# PAIN MECHANISMS
*A Physiologic Interpretation of Causalgia
and Its Related States*

# PAIN MECHANISMS

*A Physiologic Interpretation of Causalgia
and Its Related States*

## W. K. LIVINGSTON

WITH A FOREWORD BY

**RONALD MELZACK**
*McGill University*

PLENUM PRESS · NEW YORK AND LONDON

Library of Congress Cataloging in Publication Data

Livingston, William Kenneth, 1892-1966
    Pain mechanisms.

    Reprint of the 1943 ed. published by Macmillan, New York.
    Bibliography: p.
    1. Pain. 2. Causalgia. I. Title.
QP451.4.L57 1976               612'.88               76-41784
ISBN 0-306-30982-3

This Plenum Press edition of *Pain Mechanisms* is an
unabridged republication of the first edition published by
the Macmillan Company, in New York, 1943.

© 1976 Plenum Press, New York
A Division of Plenum Publishing Corporation
227 West 17th Street, New York, N.Y. 10011

Printed in the United States of America

# FOREWORD

The field of pain research and theory has suddenly come
alive—full of new concepts and therapeutic approaches. No
one in this century has contributed more to this breakthrough
than William Kenneth Livingston. *Pain Mechanisms,* which he
published in 1943, was the first major critique of the traditional
specificity theory of pain and marked the beginning of new
ideas that evolved to produce the remarkable explosion of
research and new forms of treatment that have occurred in the
past decade. Livingston exposed the weaknesses of the traditional theory, with its concept of a straight-through transmission system, and began an exploration of new concepts: the
temporal and spatial patterning of input, the importance of
summation mechanisms, the dynamics of reverberatory circuits
to account for persistent pathological pain states, the importance
of the internuncial pools in the spinal cord in the gating of
input, and the use of anesthetic blocks and stimulation tech-
niques as a way of modulating pain.

*Pain Mechanisms* is as exciting today as it was when it was
first published. The book was so far ahead of its time that few
people in 1943 understood the importance of Livingston's ideas.
In historical perspective, it is astonishing to see that Livingston
revealed and illuminated every major pain problem that concerns us today. It is a book that should be read by every serious
student of pain mechanisms in all disciplines. Its profound in-
sights in the psychological, physiological, and clinical facets of

pain make it more than just historically interesting—it is certain to stimulate and excite new ideas now as it did for everyone since 1943 who lost confidence in the specificity theory of pain and discovered Livingston's book. It provides the pleasure and excitement that comes with growing insight into a major problem. *Pain Mechanisms* is established beyond doubt as one of the medical classics of our century, and this new printing now makes it available to the wide readership it deserves.

It was my privilege to work with W. K. Livingston as a postdoctoral fellow from 1954 to 1957. It was characteristic of Livingston to seek out every possible new approach to an understanding of pain and, happily, he accepted my request to spend a year with him. The year was extended to three years—three of the most exciting years of my career. Livingston, at that time, was Chairman of the Department of Surgery at the University of Oregon Medical School. He was convinced that every clinical department should have active research laboratories so that practicing physicians and research investigators could interact, exchange ideas, and stimulate new research and clinical approaches on a day-to-day basis. He invited promising young scientists to spend a year or two in his laboratory, with the idea that they should bring their skills to bear on the problem of pain and, he hoped, continue to work on it later in their careers.

His idea was particularly fruitful. Recognizing that our knowledge of the pain-signaling system was inadequate, he proposed stimulating the tooth pulp as a source of pain signals and tracing the signals physiologically throughout the brain. Once the systems were known, he felt, their pharmacological, anatomical, and behavioral properties could be examined. As a result, a steady stream of papers on pain mechanisms appeared from the department of surgery—papers by surgeons who took time out of a busy schedule to work in the laboratory as well as by basic scientists.

In addition, Livingston organized a Pain Seminar, held each Tuesday at lunch. Its driving force was Livingston's capacity for enthusiasm and excitement. New ideas thrilled him the way new toys thrill small boys. His grin, his laugh, his enthusiasm were infectious, and the seminars covered the full range of biology and medicine. Pain was the focus of discussion, but the discussion covered all the sensory modalities, the problem of memory in all its complexity, in addition to clinical problems that provided valuable clues to the puzzle of pain. A small group, never more than fifteen people, was invited to these seminars. They included selective staff from the clinical and basic departments of the Medical School, as well as physicians from "down the hill" (in downtown Portland). The seminars were exciting, stimulating, and memorable.

Finally, Livingston established a Pain Clinic at the University Hospital—one of the first formal pain clinics established to deal specifically with pain problems that could not be solved by other medical departments. Partway through my first year, Livingston invited me to attend the clinic. "It's time for scientists to get out of the laboratory and see what pain's really about," he told me. Those clinic afternoons once a week had a profound impact on my thinking about pain. I was exposed to people suffering phantom limb pain, heard people complain despairingly of back pain and postherpetic neuralgia which failed to respond to surgery or drugs, saw people weep because of the unremitting, burning pain of causalgia. Livingston treated those patients with a special compassion and kindness, and his brilliant questions (often asked for my benefit) revealed to me what he knew so well—that prolonged pain is debilitating, demoralizing, devastating. It grinds people down and makes life a burden. People doubt themselves and think they must be crazy if so many operations and treatments do not take their pain away. And, Livingston pointed out to me, physicians in their frustration in not being able to help the patient, sometimes reinforced that view, with great psychological harm to the patient.

Bill Livingston was a big, open, warm, wonderful person. Born in Wisconsin in 1892, and raised in Wisconsin and Oregon, he received his medical training at Harvard Medical School and did a residency in surgery at the Massachusetts General Hospital. He returned to the West Coast in 1922, and set up a private practice. To get his practice underway, he acted as a State Medical Officer on workmen's compensation cases. Here is where he encountered cases of causalgia, whiplash injury, phantom limb pain, and myriad baffling pain cases that simply could not be understood in terms of the traditional textbook story of pain mechanisms. He discovered the work of Weir Mitchell, who became his model of a great physician, and he knew all of Weir Mitchell's written medical work almost by memory. When World War II broke out, Livingston joined the Navy and soon reached the rank of Commander. He requested work on peripheral nerve injury, and soon became Head of the Oakland Naval Hospital's division on peripheral nerve injuries. He had written a book, *The Clinical Aspects of Visceral Neurology,* in 1935, and steadily contributed to the literature on pain after that. All his wisdom, experience, and compassionate fascination with pain were integrated into *Pain Mechanisms,* which he wrote in 1942.

When it was first published, *Pain Mechanisms* received good reviews, but little real recognition. It simply wasn't understood. The ideas were given lip service, but the 1940s and 1950s were the heyday of specificity. Hardy, Wolff, and Goodell's book

(*Pain Sensations and Reactions,* 1952), together with White and Sweet's book (*Pain: Its Mechanisms and Neurosurgical Control,* 1955) set the stage for a powerful entrenchment of the specificity concept that pain experience is proportional to the extent of injury, and the way to block pain is to cut pain nerves and pathways. Despite the absence of recognition, Livingston persisted in his teaching, research, and writing. He knew he was on the right track, and he kept his eye solidly on what he believed was true—that pain is complex, that it is determined by interactions of inputs at all levels of the central nervous system, that it should be treated by modulating the input rather than cutting nerves. "The best neurosurgeon to treat pain," he often said, "is one with no arms." Try to restore normal inputs, he argued; do everything to break the vicious circle of pain; use physiotherapy; help the patients psychologically—in short, try every possible way to modulate activity in internuncial pools to block its abnormal reverberatory activity. This activity, if allowed to persist, will spread to adjacent neurons, involve autonomic and motor neurons, and become harder to stop in its inexorable pathological activity. Cutting nerves, he pointed out, only deprives the physician of avenues to modulate the input.

Bill Livingston's ideas, because they were so far ahead of his time, tended to isolate him. But he had devoted colleagues— Fred Haugen (anesthesiologist), Clare Peterson (surgeon and physiologist), Jack Brookhart (physiologist), and all the post-doctoral fellows who worked with him—who helped him through times of doubt and occasional despair. His greatest source of joy and support was his family. His charming, delightful wife Ruth gave him love and the kind of life he wanted to live—to work hard, play hard, and enjoy all the good things in life. He excelled in everything he undertook: in archery, horsemanship, fishing, wrestling (in his youth), and gardening. He played the clarinet well and often invited friends to play Beethoven and Mozart duets and trios. His special love of music led him and Ruth to hold their "music evenings"— listening to great music on the best equipment available at the time, and to share Ruth's superb buffet meals for such occasions.

His two sons, Kenneth and Robert, were special sources of pride. He took enormous pleasure in Ken's capacity to combine clinical medicine and research and Bob's work with Horace Magoun on the functions of the brainstem reticular formation. His wife, his children, and their families were continuing sources of strength, renewal, and pleasure for him.

After his retirement in 1958, Bill and Ruth Livingston moved to the glorious Metolius country in Oregon, where he raised plants and became an expert potter, making his own glazes out of stones he found in the area. He also wrote an enormous amount on a new book on pain he had planned and worked on for years. Pain, he argued in that work, is a trans-actional process which involves continuing interactions and feedback loops among all parts of the nervous system. Un-fortunately for the field of pain, that book was never completed. On March 21st, 1966, Bill Livingston died peacefully in his sleep.

*Pain Mechanisms* is a monument to a great scientist and human being. I recall the time when he sat in my office one Friday afternoon, as he was about to leave for the weekend. He had been writing since 5 A.M. that day—his usual routine— and decided the material was bad and had torn it all up. He was wistful and a little depressed. He wanted to know how my research was coming along. Happily, it had been a good week, and Bill beamed to hear about our new evidence for the presence of a brainstem system which exerts tonic descending inhibitory control over pain-signaling input. He was cheered considerably. "You know, Ron," he said, "Science is like a community hat into which each person contributes a little bit. Some people's work is like adding a few pennies; other people contribute nickels and dimes. Some hotshot may throw in the occasional quarter." He laughed and his eyes twinkled. "We never really know how much we contribute," he continued. "History will tell that."

History already shows that Bill Livingston's contribution to the field of pain, to the alleviation of human suffering, was very great indeed—more than he ever dreamed.

RONALD MELZACK

*McGill University*
*Montreal, Quebec, Canada*

# PAIN MECHANISMS

*A Physiologic Interpretation of Causalgia
and Its Related States*

DEDICATED TO

# RUTH

# CONTENTS

## Section Three
### INTERPRETATIONS

# PREFACE

The subject matter of this monograph has been written many times, but never in a manner that is satisfactory to myself, or to those who have an understanding of what I wish to convey. I would like to be able to present the material in the scientific language of the research worker in the fundamental sciences, and at the same time to have it acceptable to the clinician. But I find that I cannot. To a large degree this is due to my own inadequacy to the task, particularly to my limited knowledge of neurophysiology, but there are other contributing factors.

Perhaps the principal one of these is the tremendous complexity of the problems relating to pain and all sensory perceptions with which this work is concerned. To many of these problems, even the qualified neurophysiologist is unable to supply an answer. This is far from belittling the experimental investigations now in progress. The contributions from the physiologic laboratories, especially those dealing with the nature of the nerve impulse, with its transmission over a nerve fiber, or through a complex system of neurons, are of fundamental importance to the future of clinical medicine. The individual pieces of research are the building stones by means of which a new concept of the physiology of the central nervous system is being constructed. But this important work is still a long way from the stage at which it can be used to explain such clinical states as causalgia or phantom limb pain.

The experimental laboratory of the neurophysiologist and the clinic with its pain problems, have too little in common.

Even the terminology of the one is often unintelligible to the other. One has but to read a few sections of a recent issue of "The Annual Review of Physiology" to realize that each field of research is fostering its own terminology, and that unless one is constantly conversant with the literature of a special field, the current papers become increasingly difficult to understand, much less to evaluate. A further illustration of the separation between the clinical world and that of the laboratory is the attitude each has toward an interpretative concept. In the laboratory, any explanation of experimental observations which is advanced as an hypothesis, is not measured by its immediate usefulness as a concept, but by its ability to stand up as a target to be shot at by further experimentation until it is substantiated or proved false. In the clinic, an interpretation of pain phenomena is judged more leniently because it is as yet impossible to submit it to investigation under the controlled conditions of the laboratory. The hypothesis is therefore judged by its practical usefulness, and the question of whether or not it is based on a sound physiology is left for the future to determine.

It is with these considerations in mind that I have elected to write my observations and interpretations in a personal and direct manner, as nearly as possible like a person-to-person conversation, or a lecture to a class of medical students. In so doing I will venture opinions on many subjects that are highly controversial. I assume full responsibility for such opinions without claiming originality for them. It will be necessary to include some of the anatomy and physiology of pain conduction, to touch on the psychologic aspects of sensory perception, and to invade in a tentative fashion the field of the neurophysiologist. These discussions will not be treated in a technical manner, and are to be considered as necessary digressions to provide a background, rather than a foundation, for a clinical interpretation of pain problems. These subjects constitute the first section of the book. The second section is devoted to clinical cases. The third deals with interpretations.

I am indebted to many persons for assistance in producing this monograph. To none more than to Donal Sheehan, who has had a part in the formulation of the fundamental concepts as well as the actual writing of the material. I should like to acknowledge my indebtedness to René Leriche and his colleague, René Fontaine, whose pioneer work in this same field has been such an inspiration, and provided the impetus for so many valuable clinical advances; and to Joseph Hinsey, George Riddoch, Walter Cannon, Thomas Lewis, Henry Head, and so many others whose contributions have been freely drawn upon in this writing. But for my preceptor I would choose S. Weir Mitchell, who was the real pioneer, and whose observations and philosophic discussions of nerve injuries have served as the motivating inspiration for this investigation.

During the Civil War, Weir Mitchell and his colleagues, Morehouse and Keen, were given charge of Turner's Lane Hospital in Philadelphia. This 400-bed hospital had been set aside by the Government for the study and treatment of wounded soldiers suffering from injuries to peripheral nerves. The case records, the clinical presentation of "causalgia" and "reflex paralysis," which these men reported,[83, 84] and, in particular, the writings of Weir Mitchell, have never been equalled for brilliant exposition and open-minded approach to these obscure problems. With the passage of time and with changes in methods of treatment of nerve injuries since the Civil War, their contributions have been relegated to a position of historical, rather than practical, importance. Today, the single clinical

syndrome arising from nerve injury that is still associated
with Mitchell's name, is that of "causalgia." The syndrome is
comparatively uncommon, and as a result the modern surgeon
rarely avails himself of the opportunity to read Mitchell's writings. This is unfortunate, because "Injuries of Nerves and Their
Consequences" is as worthy of study as it was when it was first
published more than seventy years ago.[85]

In addition to the description of "causalgia" this text is
full of interesting case histories and penetrating comments.
Throughout the book, Mitchell emphasizes the potentialities
for harm to the individual that lie in long-continued pain. He
shows that a partial lesion of a nerve may be more capable of
mischief than complete division, and expresses his conviction
that the mischief is, to a large degree, the result of a vicious
circle of spreading reflexes, having as their source an irritation
of sensory nerve filaments. "When the later pathological
changes of an irritative nature which follow nerve injuries
begin to occur, new causes of pain arise, the reflexes become
wider, and when in certain cases the nutrition of the skin
suffers, novel forms of suffering spring up which are due to
alterations of the peripheral nerve ends or their protective
tissues."

These views, expressed so many years ago, come very close
to stating the central theme of this monograph, so much so that
I regard my investigations as an attempt to carry forward
the original work of Weir Mitchell. In actual fact, I did not
read his writings until after working for several years with the
Oregon State Industrial Accident Commission, and as neuro-
surgic consultant for the Portland Facility of the Veterans'
Administration, and at a time when a considerable portion of
my practice was devoted to the study and treatment of pain
syndromes. After this preparation, the reading provided a thrill

that nothing else I have ever read has afforded. Here, in a book by a master physician and teacher, were reduplicated my own observations, here was confirmation of my faith in the reality of "phantom limb" phenomena, and here, too, were the same speculations and groping search toward the underlying "how" and "why." My answers to these obscure queries are no more final than were Mitchell's. But if, having read this monograph, a physician acquires a more sympathetic understanding of the sufferings of a patient with an irritative nerve lesion, or a single young surgeon, disagreeing with my interpretations, is impelled to undertake a study to disprove them, then the effort will be justified.

# INTRODUCTION

In 1926, a physician, who had long been a close friend of mine, lost his left arm as a result of gas bacillus infection. The arm was removed by a guillotine type of amputation close to the shoulder and for some three weeks the wound bubbled gas. It was slow in healing and the stump remained cold, clammy, and sensitive. He sweated more from the axilla of the involved side than on the normal side, and often his shirt and the top of his trousers were damp with perspiration. At times the stump would jerk uncontrollably or, after a period of quiet, flip suddenly outward. He suffered a great deal of pain and submitted to a reconstruction operation and the removal of neuromas, without any relief. In spite of my close acquaintance with this man, I was not given a clear-cut impression of his sufferings until a few years after the amputation, because he was reluctant to confide to anyone the sensory experiences he was undergoing. He had the impression, that is so commonly shared by layman and physician alike, that because the arm was gone, any sensations ascribed to it must be imaginary. Most of his complaints were ascribed to his absent hand. It seemed to be in a tight posture with the fingers pressed closely over the thumb and the wrist sharply flexed. By no effort of will could he move any part of the hand. All the movements of the stump seemed to alter the position in space of the phantom member. The sense of tenseness in the hand was unbearable at times, especially when the stump was exposed to cold or had been bumped. Not infrequently he had a sensation as if a sharp scalpel were being driven repeatedly, deep into the thenar eminence at the site of his original puncture wound. Sometimes he had a boring sensation in the bones of the index finger. This sensation seemed to start at the tip of the finger and ascended the extremity to the shoulder, at which time the stump would begin a sudden series of clonic contractions. He was frequently nauseated when the pain was at its height. As the pain gradually faded, the sense of tenseness in the hand eased somewhat, but never in a sufficient degree to permit it to be moved. In the intervals between the sharper attacks of pain, he experienced a persistent "burning" in the hand. This sensation was not unbearable and at times he could be diverted so as to forget it for short intervals. When it became annoying, a hot towel thrown over his shoulder or a drink of whisky gave him partial relief.

I once asked him why the sense of tenseness in the hand was so frequently emphasized among his complaints. He asked me to clench my fingers over my thumb, flex my wrist, and raise the arm into a hammer-lock position and hold it there. He kept me in this position as long as I could stand it. At the end of five minutes I was perspiring freely, my hand and arm felt unbearably cramped, and I quit. "But you can take your hand down," he said.

He was prepared to submit to a posterior rhizotomy, but asked my opinion as to whether or not the simpler operation of sympathectomy might afford some relief. I was unable to predict the effect of a sympathectomy, and suggested that some time when his pain was particularly severe, a novocaine infiltration of the appropriate ganglia might provide, by its temporary effect, some index of the value of sympathectomy in his particular case. The opportunity to try this did not occur until early in 1932. On that occasion I was visiting at his home when a particularly bad attack of pain came on. We went at once to the hospital and carried out a novocaine injection of the upper thoracic sympathetic ganglia of both sides. Following the injection the stump was found to be warm and dry, and the pain in the phantom limb gone. To our mutual surprise, he felt that he could voluntarily move each of his phantom fingers. This freedom of movement and complete relief of pain persisted the following day, and when I finished my visit we agreed that the test seemed to indicate that a surgical sympathectomy should be worth doing. It was arranged that he should come to my home city in the next few weeks for this operation.

He did not come, nor did I hear from him for three months. I found then that he had remained entirely free from pain and discomfort in the phantom extremity; that the stump was no longer cold, clammy, and sensitive; and that, although sweating was present in the axilla, it was now no more than that of the normal side. He stated that this was the first time he had been free from pain in the phantom hand since the day of amputation. Though he was delighted with the result, he interpreted it as proof of the purely psychic origin of his pains and as confirmation of his fear that he was suffering from a psychoneurosis. He could not see why an injection with novocaine, the effect of which should wear off in a few hours, could possibly confer relief from pain of months' duration. I did not know "why" it could, but previous experiences with similar injections for other pain syndromes had taught me that it sometimes does confer lasting relief.

The relief from pain persisted for many months but gradually he became aware again of an increasing tension in the phantom hand and an intolerable sensation of constriction in the shoulder, as if "a wire tourniquet" were being constantly tightened, shutting off the circulation. He had been on a hunting trip in Canada about a month before I saw him in October, 1934. The weather had been chilly and, although he wore a woolen sock over the stump, it had become very cold. He believed that the exposure had aggravated his distress. At this time the stump was extremely cold and wet, measuring 10° to 12° C. colder than the same level of the opposite arm. On October 12, 1934, 5 cc. of 2 per cent solution of novocaine was injected near each of the upper four sympathetic ganglia of the left side. During the placing of the needles, as the second needle was inserted below the neck of the second rib, he complained of a sudden, sharp, stabbing pain in the base of his thumb. The needle was readjusted but the pain persisted. An hour after the injection all of the digits except the thumb felt warm and relaxed. The thumb seemed to remain pressed into the palm and was the seat of a burning pain. During the night the pain spread up the arm and he slept little in spite of heavy sedation. The following day the burning sensation gradually disappeared. The hand remained warm and the digits were freely movable. For more than seven years the pains did not return. The stump remained warm and insensitive, and there were no attacks of clonic jerking. Sweating remained normal on the affected side. There were intervals in which he seemed to completely forget the phantom arm and at times he could not even voluntarily recall its image. Within recent months, however, there have been signs that trouble might be brewing again. He has had none of his former complaints but occasionally he gets a sharp and arresting twinge of pain in the stump itself. Further treatment may yet be needed in this case.

Now let me relate another clinical history that is equally dramatic and bizarre. The patient was a young woman of thirty, trained as an x-ray technician, who complained of pain and disability in her right lower extremity since 1932. There was no clear history of injury. She was examined on February 9, 1938. During this interval she had never been free from pain but, except for short intervals in a hospital, she was able to work until the previous November. Her leg was said to be constantly cold and of a blotchy purple color. The skin was hyperesthetic, so much so that at times she could not tolerate the pressure of bed covers. She had been given a variety of treatment, including some thirty novocaine injections in various parts of the leg, mecholyl iontophoresis, typhoid injections, and various forms of physiotherapy. None of these seemed to alleviate her pain. For some weeks previous to her examination she had taken morphine each night to secure a few hours' sleep.

On the day she was examined the right leg was considerably redder than the left one, was roughened with a cutis anserina and was much colder than the left side. The coldest area was on the dorsum of the foot where the temperature measured 5° C. lower than the same area on the normal foot. The hyperesthesia seemed most pronounced here and in the popliteal space. These areas were too sensitive to permit palpation of the major arteries. Her pain could be alleviated by cutting off the peripheral circulation with pressure over the femoral artery or by using a sphygmomanometer cuff on the thigh. In carefully reviewing her history relating to the onset of her trouble, she recalled that her first attacks were always associated with an increasing sensitiveness in the upper portion of the calf muscle. An area could be accurately located in the upper, inner margin of the calf muscle about three inches below the knee joint that was exquisitely sensitive to deep pressure. In view of the failure to obtain relief by previous novocaine injections she was inclined to be skeptical about the value of further injection, but she admitted that this particular spot had never been injected. Using a small caliber 2-inch needle, about 8 cc. of novocaine was injected into this particular spot. The injection was quite painful and in the midst of it she cried out. She said she felt as if "something burst" deep in the muscle. Massage was given over the injection area and while it was being carried out the leg began to warm. The discoloration and goose-flesh disappeared and simultaneously her pain and hyperesthesia diminished. She was able to walk from the office without a limp and that night she slept soundly without a sedative. Three months later she wrote me that there had been no recurrence of her trouble. Her letter said, "I have the pleasure to report to you that I have had complete freedom from pain, tenderness, and discomfort in my leg. Surely after this length of time, the ailment, whatever it was, will not return." But it did return. One day in August, 1938, after being on her feet for some fourteen hours, she experienced transient cramping of the calf muscles. A week later she began to have pain in the muscle and down the shaft of the tibia to the ankle and simultaneously she noticed that the old "trigger-point" was again sensitive to direct pressure. She had two nights of quite severe aching pain before she reported for another injection. At this time the leg was not altered in temperature or appearance. During the injection of the trigger-point she again experienced a sharp bursting pain and within a few minutes announced that the ache was disappearing. In the next year she had two mild recurrences of local tenderness and pain, which were promptly abolished by injections of the trigger-point carried out by her local physician. Since then she has had no trouble with the leg.

Finally, here is a third clinical history. It is less dramatic than the other two but illustrates again the ability of nerve irritation to disturb the normal physiology of an extremity.

The patient was a housewife of 33, who sustained a severe bruise on the outer side of her right upper arm just above the elbow, in an automobile accident on March 4, 1941. She had an immediate wrist-drop and could not use her fingers. In the first few weeks after the accident there was an increasing sense of heat in the hand and a progressive hyperesthesia. The fingers were so sensitive that the lightest touch was intolerable and caused her to jerk away. In addition to the constant sense of burning "as if the hand were held too close to a hot stove," there was an accompanying sensation in the hand "as if electric currents were running through it." At times she experienced a similar "tingling numbness" in the tips of the fingers of the *left hand*. The extensor muscles of the right forearm had undergone a rapid atrophy and the skin over the dorsum of the hand and part of the forearm had lost its normal wrinkling and elasticity. The fingers were swollen, hot and dry, and the skin on the dorsum of the thumb, index and middle fingers was smooth and shining as if polished. Temperature measurements showed that these three digits were ½ to 1° C. warmer than the ring and little fingers of the same hand, and she was of the opinion that the contrast in temperature was frequently greater than at the time of the measurement. The hyperesthesia of the skin, particularly over the dorsum of the fingers, was so excessive that even blowing one's breath on them was painful and she guarded them from every contact. The wrist-drop was corrected and the sensitive hand protected by a plaster cast for a time in the hope that function would spontaneously recur, but the condition seemed to become increasingly severe. On June 5, the radial nerve was exposed above the elbow; at the point where the nerve passes through the intermuscular septum there was a constriction of the nerve in scar tissue for approximately half an inch. When freed by sharp dissection this segment of the nerve appeared to be constricted to about half its normal diameter. However, novocaine, and later several cc. of salt solution, injected into the nerve from below readily passed the constriction and distended the trunk to an even contour. The evidence seemed to be that the interruption of nerve conduction was due to external constriction of the nerve, rather than to scar tissue within the sheath, and for this reason the nerve was not resected but merely transplanted high in the lateral head of the triceps away from the dense scar tissue. On June 22, the cast was bivalved and the sutures were removed. Most of the hyperesthesia had already disappeared but the fingers were still very stiff and their dorsal aspects were "numb." By July 19 there was definite evidence of returning function of the extensor muscles. By August 10 she could strongly dorsiflex the wrist and could move the fingers, while the skin texture and temperature were found to have returned to normal. This woman was last examined in March, 1942, at which time she had a completely normal function of the hand and wrist and, except for an unpleasant tingling sensation, which could be elicited by light stroking of the skin over the distribution of the radial nerve, she had no residual complaints.

These three cases will serve to introduce some of the problems with which this monograph is concerned. The first problem is obvious. "Are these patients all of the psychoneurotic reaction type? Are their symptoms purely of psychic origin? Is their cure due to a form of suggestion therapy?"

Before making a conclusion that so seriously affects the status of all three patients, it might be well to reconsider the assumptions as they apply to each one. In the first place, it may be said that an inquiry into the physical and mental status of each of the three, previous to the onset of their pain symptoms, showed them all to be strong and healthy individuals who had never before showed any evidence of emotional instability, hysteria, or psychoneurosis, nor was there any evident underlying situation of "conflict." I had known the first man since we went to school together and could personally vouch for the fact that no evidences of a psychoneurosis had existed previous to his amputation. If his "cure" was due to suggestion therapy, it certainly occurred to the surprise of both patient and physician. Admittedly, it is a strain on one's credulity to believe in the reality of pains ascribed to an extremity that has long since decomposed. Bailey and Moersch [5] and many other thoughtful scientists have reached the conclusion that phantom limb sensations are purely psychic in origin and that the pain syndromes that may occur in such cases represent some form of an obsession neurosis. On the other hand, Weir Mitchell [85] never questioned the reality of phantom limb phenomena, and recently George Riddoch [102] has written a convincing and masterly argument to the effect that phantom limb pain is dependent upon some form of peripheral irritation plus, perhaps, some "sensitization" of the receiving centers. In other words, these phenomena have an organic basis. Probably the most convincing argument for the reality of the phantom limb pain syndrome is to be found in the remarkable similarity between all of the cases of this type one encounters. The larger the series of cases the physician examines, the more impressed he becomes with this striking similarity of pattern. In a subsequent chapter, the phantom limb phenomena will be discussed in more detail and this argument becomes more apparent. So, for the time-being, until a more detailed consideration of this particular type of case is undertaken, let us defer any final conclusion as to the question of a psychic or organic origin for the pain.

Now what about the second case? Here is an instance of pain of rather obscure origin associated with vasomotor disturbances and a degree of hyperesthesia that is difficult to credit. What can novocaine injected into a small area of the leg do to abolish a syndrome that affects the whole lower extremity? If it be conceded that such an effect is possible, why does the benefit persist? There is nothing known about the effects of this local anesthetic that would lead anyone to anticipate such results from its use. But is this case so different from cases of subdeltoid bursitis, tennis elbow, sensitive scar or other type of case in which a single injection of novocaine solution has been known to permanently abolish severe pain and disability? A favorable outcome following novocaine injection for sub-deltoid bursitis is less dramatic than the case under consideration, but this is a matter of degree. In actual fact, the sudden relief from pain and the almost immediate release of the stiff and resistant muscles around the shoulder-joint, which not uncommonly follow the injection of a subdeltoid bursitis, may seem almost as miraculous to the patient. In many instances the "cure" persists. There have been many explanations offered for such a cure. "The needle punctures the wall of the bursa, permitting the escape of fluid under tension"; "it opens up pathways for blood vessels to initiate a healing process in the relatively evascular fascia"; "it produces local hyperemia that acts to hasten repair processes," etc. Perhaps all of these sug-gested agencies are factors in the eventual cure of a subdeltoid bursitis, but the point I am making is that here is an organic lesion which can be treated effectively by an organic approach without invoking the interpretation of suggestion therapy. In the case under consideration it is quite possible that an organic lesion is similarly present and that the same physical agencies may contribute to its cure. However, this may not be the whole story.

The third case is the easiest of all to accept as having an organic basis. Most surgeons of wide experience have encountered a similar case and would at once recognize this one as an instance of causalgia. In this case, too, an actual lesion involving the radial nerve was demonstrated at operation and the "neurolysis" which was performed may be assumed to have liberated the nerve fibers from some kind of an irritative blockade that interfered with the normal transmission of nerve impulses.

If now, having accepted, at least on a tentative basis, these cases as having an organic basis for their symptoms, we are brought face to face with a series of questions that are most difficult to answer:

What is the nature of the organic lesion?

How can it bring about such widespread and disabling signs and symptoms?

By what means does injection therapy modify this organic lesion?

How may such a modification act to abolish the extensive disturbances of function?

Why does the beneficial effect persist?

It is only fair to the reader, to frankly say at this point that none of these questions will be given a final answer in this monograph. It is probable that neither the clinician nor the anatomist will ever be able to supply a final answer to the questions that have been enumerated. Perhaps the physiologist can do it when his investigations have progressed further. Until the physiologist accepts this challenge and can tell us the "why" and "how," we clinicians can go a long way toward establishing a practical, if not a complete, answer, and in so doing may discover methods of treatment not only for the pain syndromes under immediate scrutiny but for other disease processes as well.

SECTION ONE

# PRECLINICAL DATA

## CHAPTER I

## *The Anatomy of Pain Pathways*

It is probable that many neurons are activated between the time that a stimulus initiates impulses and the time the individual becomes conscious of painful sensation, but at least three neurons are essential to the process: (1) a *receptor neuron* (primary neuron), capable of responding to that particular stimulus; (2) a *connector neuron* (neuron of the second order), which conducts the impulses by way of fiber tracts within the spinal cord and brain; and (3) a *central neuron* in the receiving centers where perception is registered.

(1) *Receptor Neuron.*—The branching "free" nerve endings found in the skin and elsewhere are regarded generally as the pain receptors. They may interlace and overlap a wide area to give the impression of a peripheral network, but the arborizing termination of each nerve fiber, or branch of it, is generally considered as a separate unit physiologically. They are described as "bare," "free" or "undifferentiated" to distinguish them from the various types of "end bulbs," "corpuscles" and the like, of more highly differentiated sensory endings, which are supposed to subserve other sensations than pain, and which are to be found most abundantly in the skin. The activity set up in undifferentiated receptors by even a single stimulus tends to be repetitive, and there is little adaptation. By this is meant that under prolonged stimulation the receptors continue to discharge at their initial frequency, in contradistinction to the more differentiated receptors for light touch, whose rate of

discharge tends to fall off rapidly even though the stimulus persists.

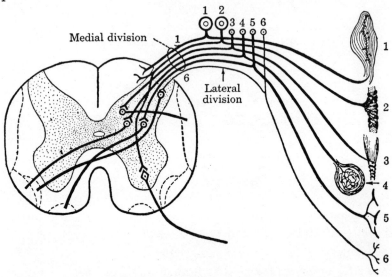

FIG. 1.—A DIAGRAMMATIC CROSS SECTION OF THE SPINAL CORD SHOWING THE PRINCIPAL SITES OF TERMINATION OF DORSAL ROOT FIBERS

1 and 2 represent large medullated fibers having large dorsal root ganglion cells and passing to the dorsal columns; they arise from Pacinian (1) and muscle spindle endings (2); 3 and 4 terminate on dorsal horn cells that cross and give rise to the spinothalamic and spinocerebellar tracts; 5, a similar cell terminating on a neuron that gives rise to the ventral spinothalamic tract; 6, a small fibered neuron (pain) terminating in the substantia gelatinosa of Rolando giving rise to a fiber of the ascending spinothalamic tract of the opposite side. (From Fulton: p. 27, *Physiology of the Nervous System*. 1938, Oxford University Press, New York.)

The cell station of the receptor neuron is in the posterior root ganglion and from here its finely myelinated or unmyelinated central process extends into the spinal cord. As they pass through the dorsal root, the "pain" fibers lie in its lateral division, which enters at the apex of the dorsal horn of gray matter. Here the fibers, each dividing into a short ascending and a short descending branch, form a small fascicle, the dorsolateral tract of Lissauer. The ascending and descending branches do not extend more than one or two segments of the cord. They terminate in the gray matter (the gelatinous substance) of the apex of the dorsal horn, where they come into synaptic relation with *connector* neurons ("neurons of the second order").

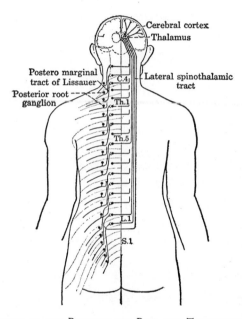

FIG. 2.—DIAGRAM OF THE PATHWAY FOR PAIN AND TEMPERATURE SENSATION

The afferent neurons of the first order ascend two or three segments in the spinal cord before making synaptic connections with the neurons of the second order. The latter cross to the opposite side of the cord and ascend as the lateral spinothalamic tract. The diagram indicates the manner in which this tract is laminated, the fibers carrying impulses from the lower parts of the body being outermost. (From Larsell: *Anatomy of the Nervous System.* 1932, D. Appleton-Century Co., New York.)

(2) *Connector Neurons.*—These secondary neurons, with cells in the dorsal horn of gray matter, cross immediately to the opposite side of the cord in the ventral white commissure and ascend in the lateral spinothalamic tract to end in the ventral part of the lateral thalamic nucleus. The fibers of the spino-

thalamic tract cannot always be traced for long distances, and it may be that part of the pathway exists as a chain of short neurons. In the cat, pain conduction through the cord is evidently bilateral and is effected to a large extent through such chains of short relays.[99] In man there may be some return of pain sensibility in the leg after complete division of the spinothalamic tract (ventrolateral chordotomy), suggesting some bilaterality of the pain pathways.

A simple plan of lamination exists in the lateral spinothalamic tract; the fibers from the sacral and lumbar segments having crossed over in the lowest part of the spinal cord, lie nearest the periphery, whereas those from the thoracic and cervical segments, having crossed higher up, are placed more deeply in the tract. The arrangement was first observed by Foerster [30] during an operation of chordotomy, when he discovered that successively deeper cuts through the ventrolateral part of the cord at the same level, raised the level of analgesia on the opposite side, step by step, from the foot up toward the level of the cord section.

(3) *The Central Neuron.*—(A) The *thalamus* is the primary receiving center for all types of sensation, the center for awareness, and apparently represents the seat of primitive emotion.

The remarkable feature of the sensory apparatus at this level is the spatial organization on the basis of an increasingly accurate representation of the body as a whole. Below this level the different modalities of sensation are distributed in separate tracts. A lesion of the spinothalamic tract, for instance, would result in the loss of pain and temperature without affecting sensations of touch and posture. Such a specific loss of sensation is not confined to isolated parts of the body, nor to the distribution of particular peripheral nerves, but instead involves the opposite side of the entire body below the level of the lesion.

But here in the lateral nuclei of the thalamus, and to an even greater extent in the sensory cortex, the different kinds of sensation are no longer segregated but are combined again into a

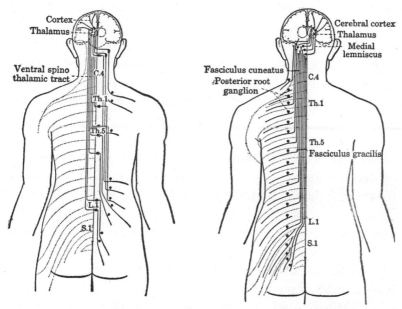

FIGS. 3 AND 4.—DIAGRAMMATIC REPRESENTATION OF THE TWO POSSIBLE PATHWAYS FOR TACTILE SENSIBILITY IN THE SPINAL CORD

In Fig. 3 the fibers of the neurons of the first order ascend the cord on the side of entrance for varying distances before making synaptic connection with neurons of the second order. The fibers of these neurons cross the cord to ascend to the thalamus in the ventral spinothalamic tract.

In Fig. 4 the fibers of the neurons of the first order ascend in the posterior columns on the same side that they entered the cord, to end in the nuclei gracilis and cuneatus. There they make synaptic connection with neurons of the second order which cross to the medial lemniscus to ascend the brain stem to the thalamus. (Diagrams from Larsell: *Anatomy of the Nervous System*. 1932, D. Appleton-Century Co., New York.)

pattern, which is not that of peripheral nerve distributions, nor of the posterior roots, but of the body units as they exist in space. So that a lesion at this level would result in a disturbance of all sensation in a particular part of the body.

Spatial representation in the sensorium suggests that the units of the sensory system remain in fixed relationship with all other units throughout their grouping and regrouping in peripheral nerves and in the spinal tracts. Such a pattern might be inherent in the anatomic arrangement of the pathways as they are being formed during embryonic life of the individual, or it might be gradually built up on the basis of experience. It is quite possible that the general pattern is laid down in the original anatomic structure and that experience merely sharpens its details.

(B) The *cortex*. The thalamus sends projections to all parts of the cortex, but the pathways subserving sensation apparently concentrate in the postcentral convolution lying just behind the fissure of Rolando. Both clinical and experimental evidence indicate that sensory functions are not exclusively confined to this gyrus, though it is the chief unit of the sensory cortex and as such reveals a very exact spatial representation. Lesions of this region disturb sensation as a whole in terms of a particular body unit, such as a leg, arm, or even a single digit. The peripheral distribution of sensory changes resulting from specific lesions of the sensory cortex therefore tend to conform to what have been called the "stocking" or "glove" type of anesthesia rather than to the pattern of distribution of peripheral nerve units.

While the postcentral gyrus is the principal center for sensory impulses from the thalamus, the cerebral activities involved in sensation are more widespread. This gyrus is in intimate functional relationship with other parts of the cortex so that all sorts of associations based on past experience may be called into play in evaluating a particular sensation. The ability to call up past experiences and judgments, enables the individual to evaluate the finer gradations of sensory impressions, to accurately localize the source of stimulation, and to make the discriminations which characterize the cerebral component of sensory experience. And while pain is generally considered a thalamic perception, an interplay between the thalamus and the various parts of the cortex takes place to modify the physical sensation.

### METHODS FOR INTERRUPTING THE PAIN PATHWAYS

From a theoretical approach it should be possible to relieve pain by a surgical attack on any part of the pain pathways. If it is impossible to remove the agent that is setting up the pain impulses at the periphery, the surgeon may elect to (a) cut the peripheral nerve, (b) cut the posterior roots over which the impulse travels, (c) cut the spinothalamic tract, or (d) excise appropriate parts of the sensory cortex. All of these methods of attack on intractable pain syndromes have been utilized by the neurosurgeon. Few attempts have been made to relieve pain by a surgical excision of parts of the sensorium, though Mahoney's [79] successful relief of phantom limb pain by an excision of a small part of the sensory cortex will serve as an illustration of this method of attack.

Although the neurosurgeon has obtained an encouraging degree of success by interruptions of the pain pathways at lower levels, this method of *anatomic* interruption is a radical and not wholly satisfactory one of treating many types of pain. It should be of value to consider some of the obstacles to success.

(a) When the source of pain lies well within the distribution of a single peripheral nerve, it should be possible to relieve the pain by dividing that nerve. This procedure has often been done and with some success. Unfortunately the overlap in peripheral nerve distribution and the spreading nature of the original stimulus combine to defeat the purpose of the operation in many instances. Another bad feature of this operation is the fact that peripheral nerves regenerate, and when the growing fibers again reach the area in which the original stimulus is still acting, the pain begins again. Most of the peripheral nerves are mixed nerves, carrying motor impulses to important muscles, and sensory impulses of touch, posture, etc., as well as carrying pain. The surgeon is reluctant therefore to cut these nerves at a high level, but on the other hand, he is aware that the closer he cuts the nerve to the irritative lesion, the sooner regeneration will be established. Furthermore, if he tries to prevent regeneration it is quite possible that the blockade will not be successful, or, alternatively, that the involvement of the growing fibers in scar may become a new source of pain.

A very similar series of problems arises when the irritative lesion involves a nerve *trunk* instead of its peripheral fiber endings. As we shall see in subsequent chapters, a lesion of this kind is more apt to cause intractable pain than is a complete division of the nerve. Sometimes the surgeon is successful in relieving pain by simply resecting the involved segment of the nerve trunk and doing an immediate end-to-end anastomosis. This method may fail to relieve the patient, or, after an interval of freedom from pain, it may recur as the inevitable scarring at the operative site causes further irritation of the nerve trunk. Peculiarly enough, Mitchell,[85] Tinel[116] and others have reported that certain instances of pain due to nerve trunk irritation have been observed, in which relief was obtained after the nerve trunk had been sectioned *peripheral* to the site of the irritation.

(b) Cutting the posterior root over which the pain impulse

travels would appear to be a much more satisfactory method for relieving pain than section of the peripheral trunks. There are two important reasons why this should be so. In the first place, only the sensory elements of the nerve are divided, i.e., the motor functions of the part are conserved. In the second place, the tendency for nerve fibers to regenerate when the nerve cell is not destroyed does not seem to hold good for the fibers of the posterior root. Once cut, these portions of the sensory neuron do not re-establish their former connections within the spinal cord. It would seem, then, that section of the posterior roots (posterior rhizotomy) would have distinct advantages over operations on the peripheral nerve trunks.

Unfortunately, the operation may fail. No matter how carefully the surgeon may have mapped out the particular posterior roots over which the pain impulses are traveling, a division of these posterior roots may not afford relief. Foerster and Gagel [29] have reported instances in which section of the posterior roots has failed to relieve the pain, but when the corresponding anterior roots have been divided the pain disappears. This would seem to indicate that the anterior roots conduct sensory impulses centrally, a view that is also suggested by the well-known fact that direct stimulation of the central end of a cut anterior root may be painful. Such evidence is impressive, but it cannot be accepted as proving a centripetal conduction of pain in the anterior roots, because the section of these roots also interrupts sympathetic preganglionic fibers whose influences may have contributed to the causation of the pain. The fact that direct stimulation of cut anterior roots causes pain may be explained by the fact that fibers from posterior root ganglion cells which supply the spinal meninges, also send branches out along the anterior roots. So that the pain may be due to activation of normally situated sensory neurons. It has been shown, for animals at least, that all pain reactions due to stimulation of anterior roots will disappear when a sufficient number of posterior roots have been sectioned.

Even an extensive posterior rhizotomy does not always abolish the pain. One reason for this is that although the posterior root pathways from one area have been sectioned, pathways from adjacent areas which previously were subsidiary in the production of the pain, may now dominate the picture. It is almost impossible for a surgeon to predict how extensive these secondary pathways may be. In addition, it is my opinion that the impulses from a focus of peripheral irritation may set up a central disturbance, probably at spinal levels, which may persist even when all possible connections between the irritable focus and the cord have been severed. This possibility will receive further consideration in subsequent chapters.

(c) Anterolateral chordotomy consists in a selective division of portions of the spinothalamic tract at appropriate levels. This operation has certain advantages over those previously mentioned. One of the most important of these is that it interrupts only those impulses concerned with the sensations of pain and temperature, leaving undisturbed the other ascending sensory tracts which subserve sensations of touch, posture, etc. As was previously mentioned, the outermost fibers of the spinothalamic tract are found to be those which have crossed the spinal cord at lower levels, that is, those related to pain and temperature sensations from the foot. By selectively dividing the tract fibers at deeper and deeper levels the analgesia progressively ascends. The operation should produce complete loss of sensations of pain and temperature on the opposite side of the body below the level of the tract section, and, because neurons within the central nervous system apparently lack the ability to regenerate, the results of the operation should be permanent. The level at which the tract fibers are divided should be two or three segments higher than the highest posterior root which may be conducting pain impulses from the affected part. This precaution is necessary because, although most of the secondary neuron fibers cross the cord immediately, a few may cross one or two segments higher than the situation of their nerve cells. If the operation is performed for pain that is unilateral, it would be anticipated that a simple division of the spinothalamic tract of the opposite side would stop the pain. But in such cases the pain relief is rarely complete, suggesting that in man there may be some bilaterality of pain conduction within the cord. It is for this reason that bilateral chordotomy is now the usual procedure. Even after a bilateral chordotomy the relief of pain is often incomplete, and in cases which show a satisfactory degree of relief immediately after the operation, the pain may gradually return. This is particularly true when the pain is of visceral origin, and it is probable that the visceral pain impulses have accessory pathways by which they may reach the sensorium. Such pathways may be represented by relays of short neurons close to the spinal gray matter, as described by Karplus and Kreidl [58] and Davis [17] or, as Foerster [29] has suggested, some may pass upward for several segments in the sympathetic ganglionic chain before entering the cord. The gradual recession of analgesia which may be observed after a bilateral chordotomy in certain instances, also suggests that impulses, finding themselves blocked from their customary pathways, eventually find new or previously unused pathways for reaching the sensorium.

A final method sometimes used for the relief of intractable pain, consists in the injection of absolute alcohol within the spinal dural sheath. The method was introduced by Dogliotti [19] and has been used often in this country for the relief of pain due to inoperable cancer. The patient is placed on his side so that the posterior roots of the nerves supplying the affected part are uppermost. A small amount of alcohol (usually less than 1 cc.) is introduced drop by drop through a spinal needle. As it is lighter than spinal fluid, the alcohol floats up around the posterior roots and apparently affects the nerve fibers more or less in proportion to their size and the protection afforded by their myelin sheaths. Thus the unmyelinated or finely myelinated fibers are damaged by the alcohol before the large myelinated fibers are involved. This is held to account for the fact that pain fibers and those subserving vasomotor control may be damaged by the alcohol while the larger fibers concerned with touch or with motor function are not seriously affected. The procedure is not painful or shocking to the patient. He may report a tingling or burning sensation that seems to sweep over the side of the body that is uppermost, but this sensation is usually mild and transient. The chief objection to the method is lack of precision and the danger of producing injury to the function of skeletal muscles and loss of control of the sphincters of the bladder and rectum. Because of these disadvantages most neurosurgeons reserve this procedure for use only in cases of hopeless malignancy.

It is quite possible that the fact that I have been dealing with such a large number of derelict pain cases for whom no procedure is assured of success, has made me overly pessimistic. I have been increasingly impressed with the *dynamic* characteristics of pain, its urgency and its remarkable ability to find a new route when the customary channels have been blocked. Sometimes when one thing after another that I do to relieve pain has failed, there seems to be a malicious insistency about it. I feel almost that it acquires a personality, like a spoiled and stubborn child which fiercely resents interference and punishment, and deliberately goes ahead seeking means to break over restraint. And I get the feeling that if I had the patience and insight I might be able to change it in some fundamental fashion so that it would become tractable.

In the treatment of pain there should be more physiologic means for its control than a mere interruption of its communications.

## CHAPTER II

## The Cutaneous Receptor and the Concept of "Specificity"

The general concept of "specificity" of cutaneous receptors has evolved from the views expressed by Johannes Müller as early as 1826.[89] In their essence these views have come to be known as the "law of specific nerve energies." Müller was writing at a time when, according to the prevailing interpretation, the sensory nerves were considered to be merely passive conductors, transmitting centrally the physical qualities of whatever external stimulus might be applied to them. He took exception to this view. He called attention to the fact that mechanical or electrical stimulation of the nerves of each special sense organ called forth sensations appropriate to that organ, and no other. He said:[89] "Mechanical irritation excites in one nerve a luminous spectrum; in another, a humming sound; in a third, pain. An increase of the stimulus of the blood causes in one organ spontaneous sensations of light; in another, sound; in a third, itching, pain, etc.—We do not feel the knife which gives us pain, but the painful state of our nerves.—Sensation, therefore, consists in the communication to the sensorium, not of the quality or state of the external body, but the condition of the nerves themselves, excited by the external cause."

Based on Müller's writings, the law of specific nerve energies can be interpreted as meaning that particular nerves subserve special functions for which they are specifically adapted. This is obviously true in relation to the organs of special sense which

Müller had in mind in his discussions. And in the main it is equally true for the sensory nerves subserving cutaneous sensibility. The morphologic differences between the several types

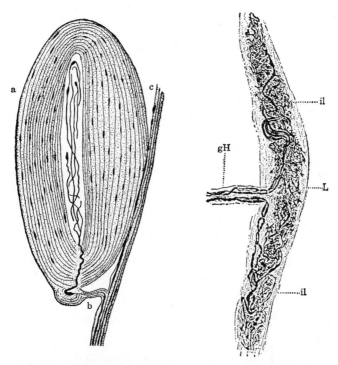

FIG. 5.—A PACINIAN CORPUSCLE AND RUFFINI'S END-ORGAN

The morphologic differences between these two highly organized sensory receptors suggest that they subserve different functions. (From Jordan: *Textbook of Histology*. 1937, D. Appleton-Century Co., New York.)

of end-organ, the variations in the size and the speed of conduction of the nerve fibers related to each type, and the distribution of sensory receptors in proportion to the kind of sensitivity shown by each part, all combine to indicate that the sensory nerves are "specific." That is, they are obviously adapted to subserve particular functions. No one believes at present that the sensory nerves are merely passive conductors, and few people are of the opinion that because an increasing stimulus may result in a change of sensory experience from touch and pressure into pain, the same sensory unit has been responsible for both the touch and the pain. It seems much more probable that the increase in stimulation involves additional neuron units whose activation contributes to the altered sensation.

Having subscribed to the law of specific nerve energies as it may apply to the sensory nerves of the skin, it remains to de·cide more exactly to what degree they are specific, and what is to be considered as the specific unit. Are there specific receptors for each of four sensations that can be derived from skin stim-ulation, and no more? What is to be taken as the specific unit: the end-organ, the fiber, the neuron as a whole, or the entire conducting mechanism for each kind of sensation? These may appear to be questions of strictly academic interest. Yet I be-lieve that they are of practical importance. Any interpretation of experimental and clinical observations must be influenced by the answer that each individual student may make to these questions. My answers vary somewhat from the answers that are commonly given, and in this chapter I wish to indicate as accurately as I can to what extent they may vary. Unfortu-nately, many of the reasons for my opinion, and the observations which have acted to determine it, must be reserved for discus-sions that will develop later. It is feasible, however, to present the interpretations that occur most commonly in the literature dealing with cutaneous sensibility, and the points which I would modify, without expecting the reader to pass on their relative merits until it is possible to develop a more complete exposition.

There are many different kinds of receptor ending to be

found in the human skin. Sherrington [107] has defined a "receptor" as a structure designed to lower the threshold of excitability for one type of stimulus and to heighten it for others. And, since the skin is subjected to innumerable stimuli of many different kinds it is in accordance with expectation to find the skin richly supplied with a great variety of nerve end-organs. The simplest form is the "undifferentiated" or "bare" type of ending in which individual nerve filaments, or free branches from a superficial nerve net, terminate abruptly without the formation of a capsule or other terminal modification. Other simple forms are the basket-ending of branching fibrils around a hair follicle, and the discs of Merkel, which are to be found abundantly at the finger-tips, in the mucosa of the mouth and lips, etc. Several of these cup-shaped discs of Merkel attached to a modified epithelial cell may form the terminals of a single fiber as it branches in the squamous epithelium. The more highly differentiated types of ending include the Pacinian corpuscles, the end-bulbs of Krause, the Meissner corpuscles, Ruffini's end-organs and the Golgi-Mazzoni corpuscles. (See Fig. 6.) An examination of these figures, or a microscopic study of a "typical" representative of each type of ending, would leave no doubt in the mind of the observer that the special morphologic characteristics of each one must adapt it to subserve a function different from that of other types. Their individual differences suggest that they are designed to "lower the threshold of excitability for one type of stimulus and to heighten it for others."

However, in any consideration of end-organ types it must be remembered that the pictures which show the internal organization of these structures are, in reality, diagrams, and that all sorts of gradations between the different types might be found in a microscopic study of human skin. In discussing the possible function of the Pacinian corpuscle, Sheehan [106] has said: "Between the largest Pacinian corpuscles that are plainly visible to the naked eye and those of Golgi-Mazzoni which can be detected only with the microscope, there is an uninterrupted

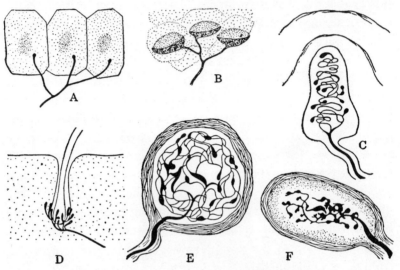

FIG. 6.—A DIAGRAM OF THE PRINCIPAL CUTANEOUS RECEPTORS

The structure of all of these end-organs is highly variable and the individual drawings are schematic. *A*, Free endings from the cornea of the eye. Note that the nerves terminate within the cell. Similar endings are found in the skin. Others terminate as networks (Woollard); *B*, Merkel's tactile disk (from the pig's snout); *C*, Meissner's tactile corpuscle; *D*, Basket-ending at the root of a hair follicle; *E*, End-bulb of Krause from human conjunctiva; *F*, Golgi-Mazzoni corpuscle from human skin. (From Fulton: p. 5, *Physiology of the Nervous System.* 1938, Oxford University Press, New York.)

series of intermediate and transitional forms. And from the so-called genital corpuscles there is a further gradual transition to the more elaborate corpuscles as described by Golgi and Mazzoni. Thus we have to remember, in ascribing any particular function to one type of end-organ, that there are all grades of corpuscle between the typical Pacinian and the other similar lamellated corpuscles."

The experiments of Goldscheider,[43] von Frey [33] and others, have shown that the distribution of cutaneous sensibility is *punctate,* so that isolated sensations of touch, pain, heat and cold may be elicited by the stimulation of discrete spots in the skin. By using hairs of varying stiffness, von Frey showed that there were special points in the skin which, when pressed upon, gave rise to a sensation of pain, quite distinct from the sensation of touch elicited by the same stimulus when applied to intervening skin areas. If a warm object of small size is applied to the skin, it is found that there are definite spots at which a sensation of warmth is experienced, and between these points little sensation of warmth is appreciated. In the same manner a cold object will register about four times as many "cold spots" as there are "warm spots." Even when an object above 44° C. is brought into contact with a "cold spot" the resultant sensation is that of "cold." By using appropriate stimuli in this fashion it is possible to map out on the skin a mozaic of spots, each giving rise to a particular sensation.

From experiments of this sort, the "punctate theory" was elaborated, whereby it was assumed that there are four "primary" sensations to be derived from the skin (touch, pain, heat and cold). Each of these "four modalities of cutaneous sensibility" was thought to be subserved by specific receptors, adapted to transmit only one kind of sensory impulse. According to this theory, pain is exclusively subserved by the undifferentiated type of ending; cold sensation by Krause's end-bulbs; warmth by the corpuscles of Ruffini and Golgi-Mazzoni; and touch, by Merkel's discs, Meissner's corpuscles and the basket-endings of the hair follicles. All other cutaneous sensations, such as tickling, formication, itching, etc., are presumed to be derived from some combination of the four primary modalities of cutaneous sensibility.

Attempts to establish an exact correlation between the mozaic of skin spots giving rise to each sensation, and the histologic demonstration of a specific end-organ for each one, have not been entirely successful. The methods that are ordinarily employed for demonstrating a skin "spot" are crude, and probably many end-organs are simultaneously stimulated. Woollard and his colleagues [127, 128, 129] have carried out intensive studies of skin innervation, and it is significant that Woollard favored the punctate theory. Weddell [123] has submitted some evidence to show that there is some grouping of "specific punctate endings lying at different depths beneath the epidermis and grouped into areas which can be defined as sensory "spots." But as will be more apparent in the light of recent observations, the histologic picture is complex and most difficult to correlate with the mozaic of spots under consideration. Differences of opinion exist as to which end-organs subserve each of the four sensations. For instance, Waterston [121] expressed the opinion that the Meissner corpuscles which are usually considered as organs of touch, may serve as pain receptors, while Fulton [35] (p. 6) says, "from Meissner's corpuscles it is impossible to evoke pain; indeed, one can insert a needle into one of these corpuscles and so cause intense stimulation without evoking conscious sensation other than that of touch or pressure." Woollard [127] favors the idea that heat and cold are subserved by specific receptors, but he comments: "It is difficult to imagine why there should be separate receptors for heat and cold since these differ only in molecular velocity." Nafe and his coworkers,[91] have conducted experiments which lead them to doubt that temperature sensations are related to specific end-organs in the skin, and they believe that "sensations of warmth depend upon the relaxation of the smooth muscle of peripheral blood vessels and the consequent pattern of sensory ending discharge," and that

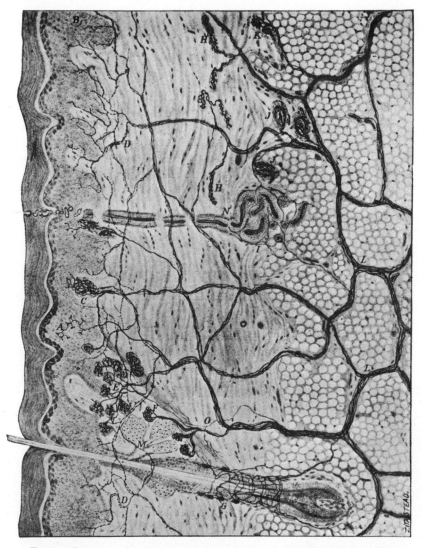

FIG. 7.—COMPOSITE DIAGRAM SHOWING THE INNERVATION OF THE HUMAN SKIN

*A*, Merkel's discs, subserving touch; *B*, Free endings, subserving pain; *C*, Meissner's corpuscles, subserving touch; *D*, Nerve fibers, subserving pain; *E*, Krause's end-bulbs, subserving cold; *F*, Nerve-endings, subserving warmth (sometimes called Ruffini's endings); *G*, Nerve fibers and endings on hair follicle, subserving touch; *H*, Ruffini's endings, subserving pressure; *I*, Sympathetic nerve fibers innervating sweat glands; *J*, Pacinian corpuscles, subserving pressure; *K*, Golgi-Mazzoni endings, subserving pressure; *L*, Nerve trunks containing thick and thin fibers; *M*, Sebaceous gland; *N*, Sweat gland; *O*, Sympathetic fibers supplying arrector pili muscle. Drawing composed from methylene-blue and reduced silver preparations. The functional interpretations above are based upon observations by the writers. (From Woollard, Weddell and Harpman: J. Anat., 1940, 74, 427.)

"sensations of cold depend upon the contraction of vascular muscles."

The highly differentiated receptor ending, such as a Meissner corpuscle, in contrast with the undifferentiated ending, is known to have a lower threshold to mechanical stimulation, and a higher rate of adaptation. The impulses which it initiates record a higher spike, and travel with a more rapid conduction rate. The morphologically complex receptor of this type is known to represent a terminal of large, myelinated fibers, while the undifferentiated type is the terminal of very small fibers, some of them having no myelin sheath. These facts have suggested another method whereby a correlation might be established between specific receptor neurons and each of the four modalities of cutaneous sensibility, i.e., by a study of nerve fiber size in relation to their physiologic characteristics.

It has been found that when cocaine is applied to a sensory nerve, its action blocks the transmission of pain sensation before it does that of touch, and it can be shown that the drug acts first on fibers of small size. On the other hand, asphyxia blocks sensations of touch before those of pain, apparently because large, myelinated fibers have a higher rate of oxygen consumption than do small fibers. The fact that different blocking agents, such as cocaine and asphyxia, acting on conducting sensory nerves, will cause fibers of different size to drop out of action in a characteristic order, has proven a valuable means for studying the conduction of impulses subserving each of the four modalities of cutaneous sensibility. In general, it may be said that touch is carried by the largest of the myelinated fibers, which do not convey pain no matter how intense may have been the stimulation of the end-organ; that pain is conducted by the smallest type of fiber; and that sensations of cold and warmth are conveyed by fibers of intermediate size. At one time it appeared that an exact correlation of this sort might be established, but subsequent investigations have shown that the correlation does not hold true.

At present it is impossible to make more than this general statement as to the specificity of fibers of a particular size in relation to cutaneous sensibility. And it is probable that the correlation cannot be carried farther because there are a number of known facts that argue against it. In 1932, Adrian [1] commented that the small fibers "cannot be classed as pure pain fibers, for they are brought into action by stimuli that would not be painful to the normal animal." He said further: "It is more likely that they supply receptors of the types suggested by Goldscheider, giving sensations of contact or pain according to the intensity of the stimulus." Pain sensation has been found to be carried not only by fibers of small size (the C group), but by fibers of the B group, and some of the smaller representatives of the A group. Warmth is known to be conducted by fibers of widely different size, varying from the size of C fibers to that of some of the fibers of the A group, not the largest of this group, but larger than those conducting cold. It is thus apparent that there is a wide overlapping of the sensory modalities through the range of fiber size, so that the fiber cannot be considered as the "specific" agency.

In spite of the lack of fully corroborating evidence to show that there is a specific relationship between each of the four modalities of cutaneous sensibility and either the end-organ or the fiber size, the general consensus of opinion seems to favor the view that there are only four "primary" sensations, each one subserved by specific receptors. And most of the emphasis is on the end-organ as the specific agent. This opinion is well expressed in an editorial on "Pain and Disease" [24] in a leading medical journal, which says: "There is still uncertainty about the anatomical identity of each of the nerve-endings in the skin which subserve pain, touch and temperature, but there is little doubt that there is in each a specific type of nerve-ending which responds to the appropriate stimulus and to none other" —and "It is quite clear that pain must be regarded as a specific sensation, and not as a mere intensification of other sensations."

The latter part of this quotation refers to the claim that is often advanced against the theory of "pain specificity," that by increasing the intensity of a stimulus, a sensation of touch apparently changes to a sensation of pain. Woollard [127] offers this anatomic finding to explain these observations. "It is a common enough observation, mentioned by others, to find a thin fiber entering into a nerve ending, a fiber quite distinct from the medullated nerve that carries the nerve ending. This additional "accessory" ending has, on the ground of its thin, non-medullated character, been reckoned as sympathetic. It may, however, and in our judgment, even more probably, be regarded as an accessory nerve of pain. It is not suggested that a receptor changed its sensation. In the eye this function is supplied by the fifth nerve, which furnishes pain receptors and pain only, to the eye itself. In the case of the internal ear the same function is undertaken by the seventh nerve. The accessory fiber exercises the same function for the hairs, Meissner corpuscles, Pacinian corpuscles and other deep endings."

One of the most frequently emphasized arguments in favor of the "specificity" of pain sensation is the fact that the central portion of the cornea of the eye is solely supplied by the undifferentiated type of nerve-ending. Since almost any form of stimulation to this part of the eye gives rise to pain, it is argued that these endings must be specific for pain. It is curious how frequently this argument is presented. I had never questioned it until, in 1931, I encountered a patient, who, after a head injury, was found to have lost the ability to respond to stimulation of his cornea with sensations of pain, but retained sensations of touch. Subsequently I have been able to test another similar case and to convince myself that a definite sensation of touch was elicited by stimulation of the central part of the cornea. When the eye was touched with a cotton wisp, the patient reported the sensation "as if you blew across the eye." The upper and outer quadrants of this man's cornea seemed to be more sensitive than the lower and inner quadrants, and in this region his report of "contact" coincided exactly with the instant of touching the cornea, with remarkable consistency. Since then I have realized that I feel the water against my eyes when in swimming, and air jets directed at the central part of the cornea without experiencing pain. And in looking up the literature on this point I found that Goldscheider and Bruckner [44] reported years ago that they had found the cornea to be sensitive to touch as well as to pain. Nafe and his colleagues [91] have convincingly demonstrated that the normal cornea is sensitive to touch and pressure as well as pain. In carrying out their experiments they used an apparatus by which very precise contact could be made with a cylinder 1.25 mm. in diameter at the contacting point, and exerting a weight of 1.5 gm. In a series of seventy-five observations on six normal subjects, the contact of the cylinder on the cornea aroused sensations of touch or pressure, but not of pain.

The question of "specificity" as it relates to cutaneous receptors becomes even more complicated when the most recent histologic and physiologic studies of cutaneous sensibility are considered. Weddell [122] has shown that the individual nerve fibers that reach a given unit of skin come to it from all directions. The pattern of their distribution is illustrated in the case of the circumflex nerve. This nerve enters the center of the area to be supplied, and breaks up into numerous bundles which proceed to the periphery of the area and then terminate as very fine branches which provide each unit of the area with the terminals of different fibers. The fiber endings that reach the central part of the area have thus traveled the greatest distance. This observation shows why, after this nerve is cut, the central portion of its area of supply is the last to regain its sensitiveness.

In the ear of a rabbit, a single fiber from the dorsal nerve breaks up into terminal ramifications which may supply many hundreds of individual hairs, in some three hundred different hair follicle groups. Presumably, a similar complex ramification takes place in the human skin, and the question arises as to how localization is possible with such an anatomic arrangement. At least a part of the answer lies in the fact that each hair is innervated by two or more separate nerve fibers whose terminals interlock one with the other. It thus follows that the power of localization must depend on the spatial summation of impulses from a number of fibers supplying the area stimulated.

Additional light has been thrown on the problem of localization and the nature of the specific sensory nerve unit, by the studies which Tower [118] has made on sensory reception from the cornea of the eye. She has found that the undifferentiated endings from a single nerve fiber extend over a whole quadrant of the cornea and spread out onto the adjacent sclera and conjunctiva. The stimulation of any part of this large unit initiates impulses that spread throughout the unit to condition each of its many parts. Apparently there is a spatial differentiation in the various portions of this sensory unit, because the lowest threshold and the highest frequency of response are obtained from the central part of the cornea, while in the outer parts the threshold is higher and the frequency is lower. This observation suggests that the stimulation of one part of a single sensory unit may initiate impulses which could be distinguished one from the other, centrally. Thus a crude sort of localization might be possible as a result of the activation of a single widespread neuron unit.*

On the basis of these histologic and physiologic investigations of cutaneous sensibility, the reason why it has been impossible to establish any exact correlation between the mozaic of sensory spots on the skin, and any single end-organ, becomes apparent. A new picture of the receptor mechanism is emerging. The individual end-organ is no longer viewed as the specific unit, but only as one terminal of a complex unit, the sensory neuron. Each unit may be remarkably diffuse in its peripheral distribution of terminal end-organs, because its fibers dichotomize repeatedly. Large, myelinated fibers branch to form a coarse mesh of smaller fibers which end in highly organized end-organs which may be as "like one another as the flowers on the same stalk." Each of these organized receptors is supplied by an "accessory" fiber whose characteristics suggest that it is related to pain sensibility. Pain is believed to be subserved

---

* Tower has summarized her findings as follows: "Putting the facts together, the sensory receptor in the cornea emerges as the terminal tissue of one nerve fiber. This is a unit, activity in any part of which, affects the whole. Moreover, there is no evidence that activity in this unit influences in any way the activity of spatially co-extensive units. Functionally, the cornea sensory mechanism appears as an aggregate of units and not as a continuum. Nevertheless, within the unit there are possibilities of correlated structural and functional differentiation such that the frequency and duration of the train of impulses conducted to the central nervous system may be determined not alone by the intensity of the stimulation but also by the site. This introduces a new condition into the central evaluation of peripheral stimulation which may permit of central analysis of peripheral locus on other than one site: 'one fiber relationship.' By central analysis of a pattern of excitation wherein fibers excited minimally, encircle fibers more strongly stimulated, a crude localization may well be achieved, yet the volume of the response from the encircled fibers, or better, the frequency of the discharge in the individual fibers most strongly excited, still serves to signify the intensity of the stimulation as has been previously assumed."

chiefly by neuron units whose fibers branch into a complicated, subepidermal nerve net that eventually terminates in multiple undifferentiated endings. The fibers of the subepidermal net seem to constitute an intricate mesh that extends over the whole of the body in a manner that suggests an intercom-

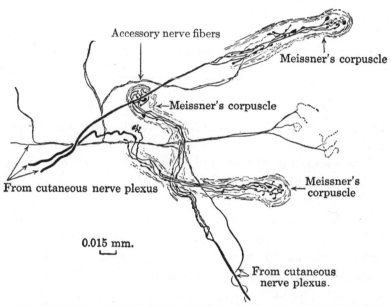

Accessory nerve fibers

Meissner's corpuscle

←Meissner's corpuscle

From cutaneous nerve plexus

Meissner's corpuscle

0.015 mm.

From cutaneous nerve plexus.

FIG. 8.—A SCALE DRAWING SHOWING THREE CLOSELY RELATED MEISSNER'S CORPUSCLES

Each corpuscle is borne upon a separate nerve fiber. Fine unmyelinated nerve fibers ("accessory fibers") giving rise to beaded terminals which ramify in the connective tissue capsule of the Meissner's corpuscles are also shown. (From Weddell: J. Anat. 1941, 75, 443.)

municating syncytium, but the evidence seems to indicate that instead of each neuron unit contributing to a continuum, it retains its functional individuality. Every unit area of skin is supplied by fibers which approach it from all directions, so that those reaching the center of the area may have traveled

the longest distance. A single unit may supply fibers to a very
large number of individual hairs, but each hair receives an
innervation from at least two different neuron units, the fibers
from each interlocking evenly around the hair follicle.

It is becoming increasingly clear that whatever the type of
stimulation applied to the skin may be, more than one neuron
unit is activated, provided the stimulus is adequate to activate
any receptor. It follows, therefore, that the impulses which underlie any sensation, no matter how "pure" the sensation may
seem to be, represent a composite of impulses arising from
more than one end-organ. This composite of impulses registers
centrally as a pattern of excitation, and from it are extracted
the sensations which we describe as touch, pain and temperature.

Sensation is a perception and as such is the result of activities
within the higher centers. It has seemed to me that in some
of the discussions of cutaneous sensibility, there is a dangerous
tendency to confuse the sensation with the mechanism that
underlies it. The danger is particularly apparent when the emphasis is placed on the end-organ, and one type is identified
with touch, another with pain, a third with heat and a fourth
with cold. The multiplicity of end-organ types, and their transitional forms, would argue against any such identification,
even if it were possible to translate sensation into terms of
peripheral mechanism. Even when the neuron unit is substituted for the end-organ as the specific unit, I find it difficult to
believe that there are four neuron types, and only four, each
of them strictly limited to subserving one of four modalities of
cutaneous sensibility. The terms, touch, pain, heat and cold,
are useful designations to be applied to sensory experiences that
are distinguishable one from the other, and it may very well
be that the pattern of central excitation which gives rise to

these experiences are customarily compounded from impulses derived from particular neuron sources. That is to say, it is probable that under normal conditions, the activation of one type of neuron may result in sensations of touch, and the activation of another type, in sensations of pain. This does not say, however, that a certain type of stimulus applied to a certain spot on the skin must, under all circumstances, result in a sensation of touch and no other sensation. I believe that the eventual sensation resulting from peripheral stimulation can be modified by changes in the peripheral environment, alteration in the status of the receiving centers, and probably by influences exerted on the train of impulses anywhere along their route from the skin to the brain. It should be possible to make this view more clear in subsequent chapters, and to indicate more definitely what interpretation may be made of "specificity" of sensory neuron units, in place of restricting their specificity to "four modalities of cutaneous sensibility."

## CHAPTER III

## *The Physiology of Pain*

Pain has been defined by Sherrington [107] as "the psychical adjunct of an imperative protective reflex." In this definition it will be noted that the protective reflex is the primary response to harmful stimuli, and that pain is the "adjunct" or the added signal in consciousness accompanying the reflex. This concept is in conformity with the generally accepted view of the evolution of protective mechanisms, in which the reflexes are held to represent the most primitive protective reaction, appearing in the scale of evolution long before any such specific sensation as pain has evolved from the more primitive affective states. Herrick [51] writes: "Our own view is that pleasurable and unpleasant experiences are not true sensations, that in the history of the psycho-genesis of primitive animals a diffuse, unlocalized affective experience of well-being or malaise probably antedated anything so clearly analyzed as the sensation with specific references, and that, parallel with the differentiation of true sensations of touch, temperature and so on in consciousness, pain sensations emerged out of the diffuse affective experience, and took their place among other qualities."

The evolutionary character of pain as a protective mechanism is indicated by the distribution of its peripheral receptors. The hollow viscera, for example, are provided with pain receptors that are fewer in number than those found in the skin, and whereas the pain receptors of the hollow viscus are activated by one principal type of stimulus, that of tension, the receptors in the skin respond to chemical and thermal stimuli as well as to a wide variety of mechanical stimuli. These facts suggest that in the process of evolution the functional units subserving pain have been distributed through the body, and have acquired the ability to respond to particular stimuli, more or less in proportion to the needs of each part for protection against the most frequently recurring threats to the integrity of that part. By countless repetition of harmful stimuli of different types applied to the exposed surfaces of the body, the skin has acquired many receptor units capable of responding to different stimuli. This defensive function of pain has been no more admirably illustrated than by Hilton[52] in his classical work on "Rest and Pain." His thesis that pain, accompanied by protective muscular spasm, is Nature's "warning signal," forms the basis on which pain is interpreted as a conservative and beneficent mechanism. Unfortunately, however, pain does not always stop, once it has accomplished its defensive purposes. And, as will be emphasized in subsequent chapters, when pain exceeds its protective function it becomes destructive.

The speed of conduction in nerve fibers of different size has an interesting bearing on pain phenomena. There is a remarkably exact relationship between fiber size and the rate of conduction of nervous impulses. The largest myelinated fibers of the human body measure some 20 microns in diameter, and they conduct impulses at a rate of approximately 100 meters per second. The fibers which have been classified as belonging to Group A, vary in diameter from this large size down to a single micron, and their speed of conduction may be anywhere between 5 and 100 meters a second. The smallest, unmyelinated fibers conduct at rates as slow as 0.5

meter per second. Those classified as belonging to Group C include these unmyelinated fibers and the smallest of the myelinated fibers, but the conduction rate for the group as a whole is less than 2 meters per second. The fibers classified as Group B tend to overlap the other groups both as to fiber size and rate of conduction. They are all less than 3 microns in diameter and their conduction rates vary between 3 and 14 meters per second.

TABLE I

PROPERTIES OF THREE GROUPS OF MAMMALIAN NERVE FIBERS (FROM GRUNDFEST, ANN. REV. PHYSIOL. 2: 213, 1940)

| GROUP | A | B | C |
|---|---|---|---|
| Diameters of fibers, μ | 20 to 1 | < 3 | Unmyelinated |
| Conduction velocity, m.p.s. | 100 to 5 | 14 to 3 | < 2 |
| Spike duration, msec. | 0.4 to 0.5 | 1.2 | 2.0 |
| Negative after-potential | | | |
| _Amount_, per cent of spike | 3 to 5 | none | 3 to 5 |
| _Duration_, msec. | 12 to 20 | | 50 to 80 |
| Positive after-potential | | | |
| _Amount_, per cent of spike | 0.2 | 1.5 to 4.0 | 1.5 |
| _Duration_, msec. | 40 to 60 | 100 to 300 | 300 to > 1000 |
| Absolutely refractory period, msec. | 0.4 to 1.0 | 1.2 | 2.0 |
| Period of latent addition, msec. | 0.2 | 0.2 | 2.5 |
| Order of susceptibility to asphyxia | + + | + + + | + |

As was previously mentioned, pain impulses may be conducted in the smaller sized fibers of Group A, those of Group B, as well as C. This would indicate that pain may be conducted by fibers from the smallest size to fibers of 5 microns or more in diameter. Correspondingly, the rate of conduction of pain impulses might vary from a half meter up to some thirty meters a second. Hence it would be anticipated that when a strong stimulus is applied to the body surface so as to initiate impulses in different types of pain conducting fiber, separate trains of impulses would travel centrally, but each at its own rate, so that when they reached the sensorium, distinct sensations of pain would be experienced. This anticipation is confirmed by many clinical observations. As an example, a man carrying an armful of wood, drops a stick so that it bounces off the end of his great toe. He experiences an instantaneous, vivid flash of pain ascribed to the point of impact, and then, after an appreciable interval, a second reverberating aching type of pain that involves the whole toe or spreads to the foot.

It is customary now to speak of "fast" pain and "slow" pain to designate their difference in speed. Anyone who has been burned, or bumped his shin against a chair, will have experienced the sharp and localized "fast" pain, then the interval in which it seems for an instant that the pain has passed by, and then the lingering aching and throbbing agony of the "slow" pain. The difference in the qualities of the two kinds of pain is just as characteristic as their different rates of conduction. The fast pain sensations are more vivid, less persistent and more readily localizable. The slow pain is diffuse, difficult to localize exactly, reverberating, and impels its victim to squeeze or rub the affected part. There are other illustrations of the slow type of pain. It has long been recognized that in some cases of tabes dorsalis there is a "delay" in the perception of painful stimulation. Pochin [97] has studied this "delayed pain perception" of tabetic patients, and has demonstrated that the time factor corresponds with the known conduction rate of C fibers. It is his view that the syphilitic lesions in some way interfere selectively with the conduction of sensation in the larger fibers of the posterior roots without preventing the passage of pain impulses conveyed by C fibers.

### ELECTRICAL CHANGES DURING NERVE CONDUCTION

It is beyond the scope of this monograph to enter into any detailed description of the laboratory methods for a study of nerve conduction. Doubtlessly, what I shall have to say about them will appear needlessly simple to those readers familiar with this field of investigation. But some readers may not be familiar with the terms and concepts in common use by the neurophysiologist, and since I shall use some of these terms in subsequent sections, I feel the necessity of making their meaning as clear as possible. Yet I find that it is difficult to define any of them except in relationship to the experimental data that suggested their use. So I am including a few paragraphs that deal with laboratory investigations of nerve conduction, for one purpose only, that of introducing a few terms and physiologic concepts which I wish to use again.

At the instant an impulse passes a given point on a nerve fiber, an oscillation of electrical potential takes place. The actual amount of electrical change taking place is so minute that only the most delicate of recording instruments are capable of recording it. With the modern cathode ray oscillograph it is possible to visualize and photograph the action potentials as they pass over nerve fibers, and to measure with great accuracy the time factors and the quantities of electrical change. By changing the speed of recording and the resistance of the circuit it is possible to analyze the action potentials of many fibers of a sensory nerve recorded simultaneously, or to study the action potential of a single fiber.

In the first type of experiment, a single stimulus is applied to a sensory nerve, such as the saphenous, and by varying the strength of the stimulating shock, to initiate impulses in a few or all of its fibers. The recording electrodes are placed at a known distance from the point of stimulation. Since fibers of different size conduct their impulses at quite different rates the photographic record will show a series of potential changes

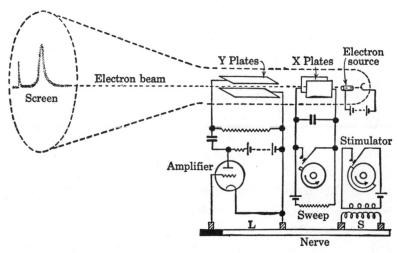

FIG. 9.—SIMPLIFIED DIAGRAM OF APPARATUS USED IN RECORDING POTENTIALS IN NERVES BY MEANS OF STIMULATOR, AMPLIFIER AND CATHODE RAY OSCILLOGRAPH

In the oscillograph tube an electron source produces an electron beam which is brought to a focus at some point on the fluorescent screen and may be viewed or photographed as a spot of light. A potential difference between the two Y plates causes the spot to shift vertically, and between the X plates horizontally. When the sweep cam opens the key, the spot, starting from the left of the screen, moves to the right at a certain velocity. The stimulator cam, which is mechanically coupled to the sweep cam, opens the stimulator key an instant later, thus stimulating the nerve through the electrodes, S, and at the same time creating an electrical disturbance, known as the shock artifact, which produces a small upward deflection of the spot. When the nerve impulse passes the proximal lead electrode, L, the amplified action potential causes an upward deflection of the spot which rises to a maximum and then declines. The impulse does not reach the distal lead electrode since it is on a killed portion of the nerve, so the action potential is monophasic. (From Erlanger and Gasser: *Electrical Signs of Nervous Activity.* 1937, Univ. of Pennsylvania Press, Philadelphia.)

representing a composite of the electrical changes in all of the discharging fibers. If the shock intensity is sufficient to activate all of the sensory fibers, it is found that the action potentials tend to group themselves into three different elevations that show a striking difference in voltage, and which tend to become farther and farther apart as the recording electrodes are moved away from the point of stimulation. These major elevations are called A, B* and C, and represent respectively the composite action potentials of fibers of the A group, the B group and the C group. By recording at known distances from the point of stimulation it is possible to measure the exact rate of conduction of each type of fiber.

In discussing the A, B and C elevations as taken from the saphenous nerve, Gasser [40] has said: "The fastest afferent impulses travel about 120 meters per second, a speed comparable to what would be expected of a good aeroplane; but fibers carrying impulses at such speeds are not found in the saphenous nerve. The highest speed sensory fibers, together with others of lower velocity—go to muscle; so the fastest component of the first elevation of the saphenous nerve has a velocity of around 90 meters per second. Other components of the first elevation grade down to 30 meters per second. Then the second sharp elevation occurs, made up of components whose maximum velocity is about 25 meters per second—equivalent to express train speed—and whose minimum velocity is about 15 meters per second. After an interval the third major elevation appears, made up of velocities of 2 to 1 meters per second. There is thus a hundredfold variation in the speed of conduction, the lowest one being no faster than a man could easily walk."

In this example of the action potentials recorded from the saphenous nerve of the cat, the actual recordings are shown in the inset figures numbered 1 to 6. The legend accompanying the figure explains the conditions under which these recordings were made. The important part of the figure is the

* More recently the B elevation is recognized only in visceral nerves and the elevation here termed "B" is now called "delta."

diagrammatic representation of the three elevations so as to show the relationship between the millivolts recorded by each group of discharging fibers and the time relation in their successive arrival at a point just five centimeters from the point of stimulation.

In another type of experiment it is possible to record the

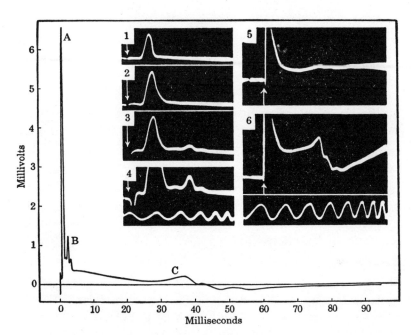

FIG. 10.—CHART SHOWING ELEVATIONS OF ACTION POTENTIAL OF THE SAPHENOUS NERVE OF THE CAT

The constituent elevations are all drawn in their proper potential and time relations from the cathode ray oscillograph records (1-6) shown in the inset.

*Inset:* Six records showing action potentials recorded when impulses have been conducted 5 cm. from the point of stimulation. 1, 2, 3, 5, 6 produced by shocks of increasing strength; *1*, fastest fibers of the A elevation only; *2*, whole A elevation; *3*, A and B elevations; *4*, same as *3* but at higher amplification to bring out the B elevation. Time for *1*, *2*, *3* and *4*, 1,000 cycles per sec.; *5*, at threshold of the C elevation; *6*, C elevation maximal. In *5* and *6* amplifications are 10 times that used for records *1-3*; time 60 cycles per sec. Time of stimulation shown by arrows. (Modified by Bard from Gasser: Chapter 11 in *Sensation, Its Mechanisms and Disturbances.* 1936, The Williams and Wilkins Co., Baltimore.)

action potential of a single nerve fiber. This can be done by stimulating a single sensory end-organ, or by successively dividing a nerve bundle until only one fiber remains functioning. If an A fiber is used in the experiment, the passage of the impulse is indicated by a sharp "spike," followed by a series of minor fluctuations in the electrical potential of the fiber before it finally reaches its original resting stage. The time interval required for the recording of the spike of the A fiber is only 0.4 msec.; whereas the interval required by the fiber to reach its former equilibrium is approximately 100 msec. During this relatively long interval, slight changes in the potential indicate that in the wake of the impulse itself, readjustments within the fiber are still taking place. Such minor fluctuations are known as "after-potential" and while they persist, the fiber exhibits an altered susceptibility to further stimulation.

After-potentials are dependent upon many factors; the fiber size, its previous state of activity, and both physical and chemical changes in its environment. In general, two characteristic phases are discernible, the first being a "negative after-potential," occupying about 15 msec. of the recovery period (for A fibers) and a subsequent "positive after-potential" of some 80 msec. in duration. A phase of negative after-potential apparently is lacking in the action potentials taken from B fibers, but can be demonstrated for fibers of both the A and C groups, although both it and the positive after-potential are subject to considerable variation as a result of environmental changes which hasten or delay the fiber recovery from previous activity.

The most interesting fact about these fluctuations in potential that follow the discharge of a nerve fiber, is that their duration corresponds exactly with the previously known ability of nerve fibers to respond to a second stimulation. Thus, an A fiber is completely refractory to further stimulation for an interval of

0.4 msec. (the "spike" interval). It is known that following this completely refractory period there is an interval of some 15 msec. during which this same fiber remains more than usually susceptible to a second stimulation. In other words, for an appreciable interval the fiber remains "supernormal" in that it is capable of responding to a second stimulus of less than the usual threshold intensity. This phase of supernormalcy is found to correspond exactly to the period of negative after-potential. Finally, after the period of supernormalcy has passed, the fiber exhibits a subnormal excitability which persists for some 80 msec. before the fiber will again respond to a threshold stimulus. This interval corresponds to the phase of positive after-potential. It is thus clear that the readjustments within the fiber that must take place after every discharge, affect its ability to respond again, and that anything which tends to alter its rate of recovery will exert an influence on its subsequent activity.

The demonstration of after-potentials has had a profound influence on physiologic interpretations. Not only has it accounted for previous observations that were otherwise inexplicable, but it has emphasized the importance of time factors in the functioning of nerves. It has shown why a nerve fiber is "conditioned" by its previous state of activity, so that for an appreciable interval it may be able to respond to less than a threshold stimulus, and for a still longer period it may fail to respond to a stimulus which ordinarily would initiate an impulse. It demonstrates why, after activity produced by tetanizing shocks, or in an environment that delays fiber recovery, the subnormal phase is "summated" and for a prolonged period the fiber remains relatively refractory to further stimulation.

The fact that a stimulus is not sufficient to initiate an impulse in a neuron does not mean that no changes have taken place in its equilibrium. A subthreshold stimulus alters the potential of the part of the neuron to which it is applied so as to render it more susceptible to stimulation. This "local effect" does not extend far along the neuron from the point of stimulation, and after an interval it dies away; but if, during the period in which the local effect still persists, a second subthreshold stimulus is applied, it may prove adequate to set up an impulse. In this manner, subthreshold stimuli may "summate" to produce an impulse in a neuron unit.

These observations taken from peripheral nerve fibers have been of great assistance in interpreting what goes on within the central nervous system. Once the nerve impulse reaches the spinal cord, or any other part of the central nervous system, it enters into possible functional relationships with a large number of other neurons, and it would be expected that oscillographic recordings taken from the spinal cord or brain would be too complex for analysis. It is true that action potentials taken from the spinal cord are complex; indeed, if the electrodes are moved from one position to another a few millimeters away, quite different recordings may be obtained. But with the knowledge gained from a study of action potentials in nerve fibers, it has been possible to learn a good deal of what goes on within the cord.

A study of "cord potentials," that is, action potential records taken directly from the spinal cord, has thrown light on many problems in neurophysiology, but in particular it has assisted in understanding what is called "after-discharge." This term refers to the relatively prolonged effect produced on the activity of anterior horn cells by a single afferent stimulus. For instance, a single afferent volley which is sustained for only 2 msec. will cause a discharge of impulses from the anterior horn which persists for 20 msec. or longer. A cord potential taken at the same time the after-discharge is being measured, will show an initial spike, followed by a double wave of negative potential which persists for 20 msec. or longer. In other words, the persistence of the after-discharge corresponds exactly with the length of time that the negative potential within the cord is sustained. From this and other confirmatory evidence, it

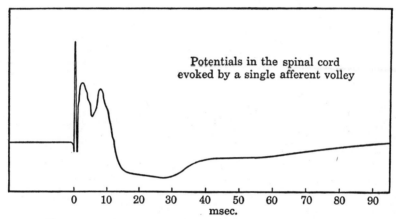

Potentials in the spinal cord
evoked by a single afferent volley

FIG. 11.—CORD POTENTIAL EVOKED BY A SINGLE VOLLEY IN DORSAL ROOT FIBERS

Leading-off electro... on surface of cord. Upward deflection indicates negativity in active region. Appearing in order are (1) an initial negative spike; (2) a much more prolonged negative potential which as is usually the case, shows two irregular waves, and (3) a relatively large and long positive potential. (From Erlanger and Gasser: *Electrical Signs of Nervous Activity.* 1937, Univ. of Pennsylvania Press, Philadelphia.)

has been concluded that the negative cord potential represents a sustained activity within "internuncial" neurons, that is, a group of spinal cord neurons interposed between the afferent and efferent units taking part in reflex activity. This group of interposed neurons, which provides a variety of pathways whereby an incoming impulse may reach the motor horn cells, has been called the "internuncial pool." The pool provides for both temporal and spatial dispersion of impulses, so that, in-

stead of a sudden short burst of activity affecting a few motor
horn cells, there can take place a sustained barrage of
these cells by impulses reaching them over pathways of un-
equal length.

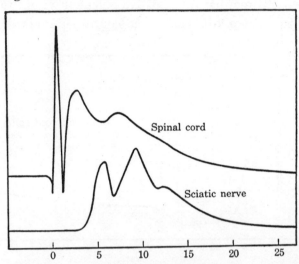

Fig. 12.—Comparison of the Duration of the Discharge of Motor Impulses
into the Sciatic Nerve with the Duration of the Negative Part of the
Potential Evoked in the Internuncial Neurons of the Spinal Cord by a
Single Afferent Volley from a Dorsal Root.

The experiment was performed on a cat under light ether anesthesia. (From
Erlanger and Gasser: *Electrical Signs of Nervous Activity*. 1937, Univ. of Pennsylvania Press, Philadelphia.)

It is probable that the number of neurons constituting an
internuncial pool is large, and that the pathways by which
the impulse is dispersed may be short and direct, or long and
complex. Two possible forms of neuron linkage have been
proposed to account for sustained activity within the internuncial pool. In Fig. 13 the diagram labelled M represents the
"open-chain" type of neuron linkage whereby impulses could
be delivered to the motor horn cells at high frequencies for
brief periods of time. The diagram labelled C represents a

"closed-chain" linkage in which the neurons could re-excite one another and thus maintain activity for more prolonged periods. This type of chain is said to be "self-reëxciting," in that activity may be sustained within the pool by impulses that

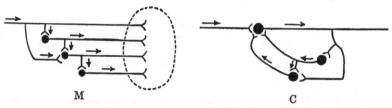

M                                        C

FIG. 13.—DIAGRAMS OF TWO TYPES OF CHAINS FORMED BY INTERNUNCIAL NEURONS

*M*, multiple chain, and *C*, closed self-reëxciting chain. (From Lorente de No: J. Neurophysiol. 1938, *1*, 207.)

can circle back through the closed chain. In such a self-reëxciting system of neurons, particularly one made up of a large number of neuron units, it is conceivable that a single afferent impulse might set up a more or less automatic activity to be sustained for long periods.

One other fact concerning the activity of the neurons of the internuncial pool should be stressed. Bard [6] (p. 106) has written: "Internuncial bombardment, be it understood, may produce either repetitive discharges in motor neurons by delivering impulses of threshold density or it may subject the motor neurons to rapidly repeated subliminal rises in excitability by impulses which are not dense enough to cause threshold excitation. The latter effect is important because it will facilitate any intercurrent stimulation." In other words, activities within the internuncial pool, even if they are not sufficient to cause muscular contraction, may render the motor horn cells unusually susceptible to any intercurrent stimulation. This is hardly the place for speculative discussion of clinical observations, but I am impelled to wonder if some such mechanism as this may not underlie the heightened reflexes, the excessive responses to noise, and perhaps the clonic jerking of a stump, which have been observed in patients who have long suffered from a continuous train of afferent impulses of painful intensity.

The concept of an internuncial pool of neurons within the central gray matter, that are interposed between receptor neurons and effector units, has been of great assistance in understanding the activities that characterize the central nervous system as a whole. For instance, it has long been known that a first "conditioning" volley of afferent impulses increased the magnitude of response to a second "testing" volley. The greater reflex effect of the testing volley can be explained as due to the arrival at the motor horn of some of its impulses, coincident with the arrival of impulses set up by the conditioning volley which have been delayed in reaching the anterior horn cells by passing through longer chains of the internuncial pool. This phenomenon of "facilitation" is one of the characteristics of central nervous system function and is dependent upon a temporal dispersion of impulses within the internuncial pool which favors the response to, or augments the effects of, newly arriving impulses.

Another characteristic of central nervous system function is that of "inhibition." There are probably different kinds of central inhibition, none of them well understood, but the concept of the internuncial pool has been utilized to illustrate certain forms of inhibition. But whether the internuncial pool concept is sufficient alone to explain central facilitation and inhibition, there can be no doubt that both of these active processes are constantly exerting an effect on all incoming sensory impulses. Head [49] reached the opinion, many years ago, that the neurons of the posterior horns of the spinal cord were more than simple relay stations. He believed that they were capable of either facilitating or inhibiting the sensory impulse before it reached the secondary neuron, and that they were actively engaged in integrative functions affecting all normal sensory impulses. And it was his view that this central integration was not confined to the spinal segment at which the sensory impulse entered the cord, but continued to modify the pattern of impulses at each functional level between the spinal segment and the sensorium. He said [46] (p. 832): "Our conception of the mechanism of somatic sensitivity is fundamentally opposed to all previous psychological and physiologic teaching. We believe that the physical forces of the external universe produce within us a number of impressions, which are in many cases incompatible with one another from the sensory point of view. These are sorted, combined and controlled within the central nervous system until they are sufficiently integrated to underlie sensation; the final product being simpler than its constituent elements. There are no physiological activities corresponding to 'primary' sensation. The afferent impressions produced by the actions of an external stimulus are highly complex, and are subjected to the integrative action of the central nervous system, before they can become fitted to subserve sensation. Qualities such as pain, heat and cold are abstracted from the psychical response and spoken of as 'primary sensations;' but they have no physiological equivalent in the vital reactions of the peripheral mechanism. A 'primary sensation' is an abstraction. Afferent physiological processes are most complex at their origin; they become continuously more specific and simpler as they are subjected to the modifying influence of the central nervous system."

I am entirely in sympathy with this view, and will amplify Head's concept in the next chapter, but for the moment the point under consideration is how pain impulses may be modified by intraspinal activity. It has been suggested that the discriminative sensations—touch, posture, etc.—normally exert an inhibitory influence on the impulses subserving pain, so that unless these impulses are so strong as to dominate the entire sensory pattern, the sensation of pain, as such, does not register in consciousness. If all stimuli above a certain intensity were to be permitted to call forth involuntary protective reactions, (and incidentally to be felt as pain sensation), learning processes would be made difficult, discriminative reactions interfered with, and the efficiency of the individual would be seriously curtailed. Therefore, under normal conditions the central activity tends to favor the transmission of the discriminative sensibilities and to inhibit pain impulses. Under abnormal conditions, such as involves a distortion of normal relationship, the pain pathway is thrown wide open and the passage of impulses by this route is facilitated. An abnormal situation of this kind apparently results in certain instances of injury involving the posterior columns, lesions of the central gray matter, and when long-continued and dominating impulses of painful intensity assault the central nervous system.

This view is of necessity an interpretation, and has never been experimentally corroborated. But there is experimental evidence for the existence of an internuncial pool in which just such modification of sensory impulses might take place. In discussing the influence which the internuncial pool may exert on afferent impulses, Gasser [39] has said: "A given stream of afferent impulses over a peripheral nerve follows one pathway in the centers at one time and another pathway at another time. The direction of the switching is conditioned by the situation obtaining at the moment, and is always consonant with a coordinated reaction of the whole organism"—and— "Anatomical peculiarities of the form and arrangement of endings differentiate the ease of transmission spatially, and the nature of the previous activity differentiates it temporally"— and, again—"Ultimately, excitation in a pool of neurons is dependent upon everything which is taking place in the nervous system anywhere because of the direct representation of this activity in the population of endings in the pool."

In closing this chapter I should like to add a personal comment. I was brought up in a medical generation in which the "reflex arc" of two, or possibly three neuron units, was not interpreted as a symbol of a very complex function, but as an actuality. I received the impression that pain was a primary sensation, dependent upon the stimulation of a specific sensory ending by a stimulus of a certain intensity, and conducted along a fixed pathway to ring a special bell in consciousness. Pain was as simple as that, and to me the pathway was as immutable and inevitable as the overhead wires in the "General Store" which conveyed baskets to the cashier's desk. The idea that anything might happen to sensory impulses within the central nervous system to alter their character, destination, or the sensation they registered in consciousness was utterly foreign to my concept. But in practice, I found that it was increasingly difficult to make this concept consistent with clinical observations. I presume I was encountering the same sort of clinical problems that led such men as Weir Mitchell [85] and Henry Head [46] to rebel against the idea that all cutaneous sensations were "specific," and to recognize the psychic factor in all syndromes characterized by severe and protracted pain. At least, I found in their writings, and in the more recent papers of George Riddoch,[101] an interpretation of pain to which I could subscribe without reservation. The reader will find in these references an exposition of this viewpoint which I know to be consistent with clinical observations.

## CHAPTER IV

## The Psychology of Pain

The chief difficulty encountered in a search for a satisfactory definition for pain, is the fact that it can be considered from either a physiologic or a psychologic approach. Any consideration of pain by one approach alone, without due regard to the other, is incomplete. It cannot be defined in terms of strength of stimulus, nor the specialized units concerned in its conduction. These may be important factors in its mechanism, but they are not pain. Pain does not always accompany protective reflexes, even violent ones, nor are protective reflexes necessarily the precursors of painful sensation. Pain is a perception; it is subjective and individual; it varies in different races of people; and individual susceptibility to pain may vary with changes in emotional and physical equilibrium.

In this connection it is of interest to note that certain individuals have been found from time to time, who appear to be lacking, to a remarkable degree, in pain susceptibility. Ford and Wilkins [31] have reported three instances of this extraordinary condition in children. All three showed normal responses to touch and temperature stimuli, and two of them gave evidence that adequate stimulation of internal organs might give rise to sensations of pain. Yet deep pricking of the skin in any part of the body, strong compression of the Achilles tendon, and other forms of stimulation, usually painful, elicited neither pain sensation nor the involuntary reflexes that customarily arise as a result of such strong stimuli. There were no increases in the heart rate, no "psychogalvanic response," and no protective withdrawal reflexes observed during their tests. Ford and Wilkins were of the opinion that in their cases there was no evidence of hysteria, nor any organic deficiency in the pain conducting mechanism. Rather, they felt that to an unusual degree these children *disregarded* pain. If this is the true explanation, such an ability to disregard pain is certainly not common, but lesser degrees are seen in the disregard for discomfort and even pain, of the man engrossed in any subject that holds his emotional interest, in the Indian fakir, the Chinese coolie, and in certain religious fanatics who torture themselves.

Pain can be evaluated only by the individual experiencing it. The human animal is the only one who can analyze his sensation and describe it to someone else. Therefore the physiologist who carries out his investigations of pain on experimental animals other than man is at a tremendous disadvantage. It is true, he can rigidly control the conditions under which his experiment is conducted, and hence can rule out many of the variables that hinder an accurate evaluation of pain under clinical conditions, but he is compelled to estimate the degree of pain the animal suffers, by observing its actions. And the animal's reactions are not a reliable index of the vividness of the sensation evoked by a particular stimulus. The very nature of his investigation tends to concentrate his attention on the physical aspects of the sensation, and to permit him to ignore the apperceptions which, in man at least, tend to modify the perception.

Herrick [51] has said: "Few problems in neurology are more difficult and involved than those centering about the nerves of painful sensibility. This question is intimately related with the disagreeable and pleasurable feelings and with the affective and emotional life as a whole. Nearly all sensations, whether of the somatic or visceral center, appear to have an agreeable or disagreeable quality. There is difference of opinion as to whether any sensation is wholly indifferent in this respect. There are, however, two factors in this situation which have not always been distinguished, and whose introspective analysis is very difficult. In the first place, many sensations are, as such, painful or pleasurable, and in the second place, the related apperception, ideas, etc., may have an agreeable or disagreeable feeling-tone. The intimate relation of these two factors in consciousness probably grows out of the similarity in the type of physiological process involved in their neurological mechanisms, and this, in turn, may rest on the fact that the two mechanisms in question have a common evolutionary origin."

In every patient there are added to the sensory perception, initiated by the physical impulses registering as pain, any number of associated ideas, apperceptions and fears, the sort of fear that has been defined as "anticipatory pain," that may become indistinguishable one from the other. A painful sensation of mild degree, but of unknown origin, may become, because its source is not recognizable, associated in the mind of the patient with his fear of cancer, or a fear of death, until it is transformed into a new and unbearable suffering. On the other hand, convincing evidence that his fears are unfounded may immediately reduce the painful sensation to negligible proportions. As for the patient's own introspective analysis of his pain, he may realize that his toothache does not actually increase during the night when his dentist is not available. He may appreciate the fact that with the quiet of night other incoming sensory experiences diminish, there is less to preoccupy his mind, so that the pain now occupies the focus of his attention. As he climbs into the dentist's chair the next morning, he may know that the pain hasn't gone. But, in spite of such rationalizations, the pain seems to him to increase at night and diminish when relief is at hand, and as far as his ability to tolerate the pain sensation is concerned, such fluctuations in intensity are very real.

## THE CONCEPT OF THE "BODY SCHEME"

Even the ability to localize pain has psychologic implications. Head and Holmes [48] suggested long ago, that on the basis of sensory experience, every individual creates for himself a "body scheme," which represents the image of his body parts as they exist and move in space. This image of himself serves as the "plastic model" in consciousness by which he gauges his own movements and localizes stimuli. Throughout life, all sensory experiences, be they postural changes, touch, pain or temperature sensations, or visual perceptions, combine to slowly perfect this plastic model of self. Gradually the model assumes more exact form and with training and stored experience, it becomes the agency by means of which he projects himself as a coordinate unit. Confronted with a new situation, he does not command individual muscles to function, but instead he wills the act in terms of this image of himself. And even as he starts the willed effort, the messages that come back to consciousness, fall into place on the sensory image to tell him whether or not he is doing the task correctly. It is reflected sensory impressions such as these, evaluated against the stored impressions of the self image, which tell the baseball pitcher that the throw "felt right," and he knows exactly where the ball will go and how it will behave in its flight even before his visual perceptions confirm that impression. It tells the archer, in the instant of loosing the arrow, that it is to fly true to the "gold."

Riddoch [102] has suggested that actually there are three plastic models created at the perceptual level. The first is derived from postural sensibility and this model is essentially concerned with body movements. The second is built up by cutaneous sensations that are related to body shape and localization. The third, and perhaps the least essential of the body schemata, as far as recognition of somatic impressions are concerned, is acquired through visual sensation. Riddoch makes it clear, however, that in the normal individual the plastic model of himself is a sensorimotor unit and not an aggregate of functionally separate parts. It is only when some dissociation of sensory perception takes place that the composite parts of this whole make themselves apparent. Under certain abnormal conditions, the exact nature of which is not clear, disorders of sensory perception may lead to a dissociation of these plastic models from actuality or from one another. In certain instances, following a hemiplegia, the patient retains the feeling that his paralyzed limbs are movable. He may insist that the limbs function normally, and his illusion tends to persist in spite of visual evidence to the contrary. After an amputation, the subject usually retains a vivid impression of the presence of the lost member, and when pain impulses from the cut nerves in his stump persist, he may retain the "phantom" illusion for many years, and often is more conscious of the presence of the phantom than of his normal extremities. It is apparent that in both of these types of dissociation of the plastic model from actuality, the model has persisted unchanged while it is the body that has changed. In contrast with this type of dissociation are those cases in which there are no actual changes in the body itself, but some alteration takes place in the model. Presumably this type can occur with lesions involving the parietal cortex. According to the extent and location of the lesion, all sorts of dissociations may take place, from instances in which there are but slight distortions of sensory perception of the body, to cases in which there is loss of awareness of one whole side of the body. Nielsen [92] has reported the case of a dentist who experienced episodes during which he was totally unaware of the left side of his body. The clinical notes from this case report: "On several occasions he undressed the right half of his body and went to bed with the left side still dressed. He did not notice this until his wife called attention to it. In taking a bath, he dried the right side of the body, threw the towel over the left shoulder and left it hanging there. He then began to dress without.drying the left side." In right-handed persons, it seems that the sensory loss of one side of the body is always confined to the left side, and that only in left-handed people may the right side be lost to perception. A lesion involving the dominant hemisphere apparently results in quite a different sensory dissociation. Such an observation suggests that the two hemispheres are, in some unknown fashion, interdependent in maintaining the normal plastic model of self.

Riddoch [102] has utilized the concept of the "plastic model" to explain many of the phenomena of the "phantom limb." He has observed similar phantoms that persist after the loss of a nose, a breast or the penis. In the sensory illusion of a phantom limb, it is the parts most richly endowed with sensory receptors, and which during life have been most highly trained in both precision and sensibility, that are most clearly perceived by the subject. This implies that these parts of the perceptual image of self, have, during the years of schooling and building up of the plastic model, become most clearly defined. Thus the man who retains the impression of the constant presence of his amputated arm does so in terms of the plastic model. He is rarely conscious of all parts of the phantom limb. The upper arm may not be felt at all; the elbow is rarely perceived although it may seem to move in a normal fashion with the rest of the phantom; the forearm and wrist are apparently present in some instances; but the hand may seem more real than the remaining normal hand. A later chapter will be devoted to this subject of phantom limbs, and in it the subject of "body scheme" will again come up for further discussion.

It is not the purpose of this section to develop the idea of the fundamental *oneness* of mind and body. It has been splendidly developed in such texts as those of McGregor [78] and Dunbar,[20] and in varying degrees is a part of every physician's concept of his patient. Everyone is aware, too, of the "vicious circle" of perturbed function of both the psychic and the physical fields that may be initiated by disease or by emotional stress. An illness leads to worry, the worry in turn disturbs the smooth functioning of internal organs, which in their turn add to the burden of symptoms, and so the circle goes like a rolling stone that gathers momentum as it progresses down an incline. In combatting this progress it makes but little difference which aspect of these mutually mirroring processes is first attacked, so long as the original process that starts the cycle does not involve permanent organic changes. What starts as a functional process, once involved in the vicious circle, may eventually lead to organic changes, and this seems to hold true whether we are talking about "dyspepsia," "Raynaud's disease," or "causalgia." Even after organic change has started, a reversal of the process may lead to a cure of the symptoms and in some instances the disappearance of the organic lesions and a restoration of normal function.

The psychologic aspects of this problem, and the fact that organic lesions of the central nervous system may lead to functional disturbances, and eventually to secondary lesions of the internal viscera, are too well recognized to require discussion here. The subject is mentioned only as forming the background for a consideration of the destructive potentialities of pain.

Pain may be considered as "protective" as long as it assists the individual in avoiding harmful agencies that threaten his safety and well-being. To this extent it is conservative and beneficent, and it is this aspect of pain that has been most frequently emphasized. Unfortunately pain does not often stop when it has accomplished its protective function, and, unfortunately too, many of the painful conditions from which human beings suffer cannot be avoided or eluded, no matter how intelligent the individual may be. Leriche [64] has reacted violently against the viewpoint that considers pain as a beneficent mechanism. He says this concept of pain is "an extraordinary error—which has no shadow of justification." His book, "The Surgery of Pain," makes a brilliant exposition of the destructive nature of pain, and goes far to justify his view. Certainly it is true that when a pain is intense and long-continued, it may dominate the sensorium. It interferes with thought processes, it disturbs sleep, impairs appetite, undermines morale, and may disorganize the functioning of every part of the body. Mitchell [85] (p. 196) has said: "Perhaps few persons who are not physicians can realize the influence which long-continued and unendurable pain may have upon both body and mind. The older books are full of cases in which, after lancet wounds, the most terrible pain and local spasms resulted. When these had lasted for days or weeks, the whole surface became hyperaesthetic, and the senses grew to be only avenues for fresh and increasing tortures, until every vibration, every change of light, and even, as in Miss Willson's case, the effort to read brought on new agony. Under such torments the temper changes, the most amiable grow irritable, the soldier becomes a coward, and the strongest man is scarcely less nervous than the most hysterical girl."

## PSYCHIC PAIN

To classify certain types of pain as "psychic" pain is purely arbitrary, because all pain is a psychic perception. However, the term has been used to designate a type of pain for which there is no organic basis, in the nature of a lesion, either peripheral or central. There is a tendency, rather widespread, to use this term in a loose manner to apply to cases in which there is no *obvious* organic origin for the pain. I regard this tendency as being as harmful to the true understanding of pain as the emphasis that is sometimes placed on the theory of specificity in its narrowest sense. The easiest way to illustrate what I have in mind, is to quote a few passages from a chapter entitled "Psychoneurotic Pain" contained in a well-known psychologic text.[7]

"In certain clinical situations the purely psychic nature of pain is unmistakable. *John W.* had the misfortune to touch a high voltage wire with his open hand. The current caused vigorous spasm of the muscles which drew the hand and forearm into painful flexion. The electrical burns were so extensive that it was necessary to amputate the arm above the elbow. Following this operation there was no unusual discomfort at the stump, but the patient was distressed by the apparent contracture of the now non-existent hand and forearm. *George B's* experience was similar. He was annoyed by gravel in his glove while working on a railroad track. Before he could remove the glove he was struck by a train and his arm was crushed so that amputation became necessary. After the operation he was annoyed less by the pain of the amputation than by the feeling of gravel at the missing finger tips.

"The psychoneurotic patient may complain of pain long after surgical wounds have healed. *Mrs. Drusilla D.* continued to have rectal pain after a successful operation for hemorrhoids. She insisted that a nerve had been caught in scar tissue, and she refused to believe the numerous physicians whom she consulted and who assured her there was no physical cause for her discomfort. Eventually she became negativistic. She refused to eat because bowel movements were painful, and because she did not know what was to become of the food. She was placed under hospital care and fed by nasal tube. However, she learned to vomit the contents after tube feedings and shortly she died of inanition. This is an extreme case, but it illustrates the fact that a neurotic individual can make an obsession of pain and that the resultant mental disorder may assume major proportions.

"Not infrequently there is persistent complaint of pain after amputation of a limb. Despite satisfactory surgical results the patient complains of aching, throbbing, pinching, tenderness, etc., and he may even persuade the surgeon to explore the stump or amputate the limb a little higher. When the pain is psychoneurotic the results of a second operation are almost invariably disappointing. The situation is similar with abdominal surgery. A scar may be painful and tender. It may burn and ache. The contact of clothing may be annoying or distressing. But woe to the surgeon if he fails to recognize the psychoneurosis and if in a weak moment he consents to explore the abdomen for adhesions."

I find myself completely at variance with the implications drawn from these cases. I am not in a position to deny the possibility that in these specific instances the pain was "purely psychic," but I seriously doubt that conclusion, and I protest the implication that might be drawn from such cases and applied to similar cases which I have personally investigated. I shall have much more to say about the phantom limb syndrome, and I find myself sympathizing with John W. and George B., who suffered from it. And I am impelled to wonder if Mrs. Drusilla D., who became negativistic, and, stubborn creature, eventually died of inanition, may not have been entirely correct in her assumption that a sensory nerve had been caught in a scar after her successful operation for hemorrhoids.

My training does not qualify me to speak with authority in any part of this chapter dealing with certain of the psychologic aspects of pain, but I am sure of my ground when I warn against the indiscriminate employment of the term "psychic" pain in classifying cases that lack an obvious organic basis for their complaints, or simply because their signs and symptoms fail to conform to the generally recognized patterns of nerve distribution.

## "CENTRAL INTEGRATION" OF SENSORY IMPULSES

Now, if the concept of psychic pain as a thing apart and the theory of "specificity," in its narrowest sense, are to be discarded, what alternative concept is to take their place? For myself, I would select Head's [46] concept of central integration of sensory impulses as best meeting this need. It seems worth while to quote him once more (p. 832): "We believe that the physical forces of the external universe produce within us a number of impressions, which are in many cases incompatible with one another from the sensory point of view. These are sorted, combined and controlled within the central nervous system until they are sufficiently integrated to underly sensation; the final product being simpler than its constituent elements. There are no physiological activities corresponding to 'primary' sensation. The afferent impressions produced by the actions of an external stimulus are highly complex, and are subjected to the integrative action of the central nervous system, before they can become fitted to subserve sensation. Qualities such as pain, heat and cold are abstracted from the psychical response and spoken of as 'primary sensations,' but they have no physiological equivalent in the vital reactions of the peripheral mechanism. A 'primary sensation' is an abstraction. Afferent physiological processes are most complex at their origin; they become continuously more specific and simpler as they are subjected to the modifying influence of the central nervous system."

This quotation gives to me the essence of the whole story. Yet I find myself wondering how such integrations take place, of what does "specificity" consist if it cannot be expressed in terms of sensation, and how does sensation register at the perceptual levels. No one can give the answers to these questions, but I have tried to express my own groping interpretations to my students, and to find comparisons taken from fields with which they are more familiar, to convey my meaning.

In expressing my concept of the specificity of peripheral receptor neurons, I have compared them with radio-receivers. The Government allocates certain radio frequencies as broadcasting channels for various agencies. There are a number of these broadcasting "bands," and radio receivers could be constructed that would be specially adapted to pick up each band. Let us suppose that we have five such receivers, one for the "regular" broadcast band, one for a "police" band, one for an "amateur" band, one for a "high frequency" band, and one for the "government" band. Each receiver could be tuned to several stations within the limits of the frequencies which it was constructed to pick up. Certain of these stations might be expected to give superior reception and we might customarily leave each receiver tuned to such a station. It is further probable that the type of program or the kind of sounds we would pick up with each type of receiver usually would be characteristic of its particular band. The obvious point in this comparison is the fact that no single receiver is restricted to any single station or any particular type of program. Within the limits of the frequencies to which it is specifically adapted, and subject to tuning, atmospheric conditions and a number of other factors, its capacity for reception is remarkable for its variability rather than for its limitations. In somewhat the same way, I believe that sensory neurons are specifically adapted for responding to stimuli whose physical characteristics fall within certain "frequency" limits. It is quite possible, even probable, that these receptor neurons are capable of a certain variation in "tuning" according to their intrinsic and environmental status, and, furthermore, it is conceivable that under "normal" conditions they may be engaged chiefly in transmitting certain kinds of impulses that eventually are perceived as a particular kind of sensation. However, their "specificity" is measured only by the limits of the frequencies to which they can respond under any and all conditions.

Exactly what Head means by the "integrations" that take place to modify the sensory impulses when they reach the spinal cord and at the various functional levels below the sensorium, is not clear. But the internuncial pool concept furnishes an implement whereby both inhibition and facilitation of the impulses might take place. It is possible that under "normal" conditions the "tuning" of the internuncial activity might favor the transmission of the impulses subserving discriminative sensibilities and inhibit those that tended to interfere with the functional efficiency of the individual. Under other conditions such as might be occasioned by sustained irritations, either peripheral or central, the opposite effect might be produced. As a result, discriminative sensibilities might be suppressed, and pain dominate the sensorium.

One of the reasons I have always objected to a consideration of pain as a "pure" sensation is that there are so many kinds of pain, and so many concomitant sensations that may be perceived along with the pain sensation. In even as simple an instance as pain from a needle prick, the critical observer will find that he perceives many things in addition to the sensation he labels "pain." He can tell where it occurred, how intense was the stimulation, and perhaps even the size, shape and relative sharpness of the pricking instrument.

It is as if a musically trained individual were to hear three different instruments sound "A." He would say instantly, "That is a violin," or "That is a clarinet," or "That is a French horn," without being in the least aware of the overtones, or their relative values which combined to give the instrument its characteristic tone quality. He might be able to state that each instrument sounded "A" and that this tone had 440 vibrations per second. But that would not tell the whole story, for if the fundamental were to sound alone, the instruments would lose their identity. To tell the whole story would require an exceptionally gifted musician, who could identify each overtone and describe its intensity in relation to the fundamental tone. Even this gifted person might have difficulty in telling exactly why the tone of a Stradivarius violin was superior to that of another violin. The fact that different instruments may be recognized, not only by their overtones, but by qualities even more subtle, indicates that the listener hears a complex of sounds, even though he may be able to identify only the fundamental.

In much the same sense, the perceptions arising from cutaneous stimulation are the result of many different impulses registering simultaneously in the sensorium. We may describe them as sensations of touch, pain or temperature because one perception seems for the time being to dominate the other sensory impressions.

Much this same concept of sensory perception as being a central interpretation synthesized from a composite of many different afferent impulses and apperceptions, is beautifully expressed in Parsons',[95] "An Introduction to the Theory of Perception." His interpretations are of particular significance because they are drawn chiefly from his study of visual sensation, a sensory modality that is considered to be the outstanding example of a "specific" sensation. Certainly the visual apparatus is made up of highly specialized units subserving a single function. The receptor end-organs, the conducting pathways, and the cortical and subcortical centers subserving vision represent the most specialized sensory mechanism of the human body; in fact, there is almost point-to-point relationship between parts of the striate cortex and the retinae. The point that Parsons makes is that central perception is quite another thing from the impulses which activate it. It is his view that the final perceptual "pattern," while perhaps described as a unit sensation, is actually greater than its constituent parts and hence is a new entity. He also points out that the percepts vary with the state of the receptor organ and with the changing status of the receiving centers. He says (p. 239): "Investigation and analysis have further shown that we cannot experience a pure, isolated sensation. We can reduce the variables to a minimum and then proceed to apply an adequate stimulus to a given receptor and study the results. Such experiments have afforded highly valuable results, but they have also conclusively shown that the results depend not only on the stimuli and the state of the receptor organs, but also on the state of the central affector organs, the conducting paths being the most stable part of the system. They have further shown that the functional activity of the central organs is modified by a multitude of factors, especially the results of previous excitation and the backstroke influence of higher centres."

Lashley [63] has carried out an important series of studies dealing with the functions of the visual cortex in rats. Some of his observations are most difficult to explain on the basis of the generally accepted ideas of the specificity of function of particular neurons of the visual cortex. For instance, if a rat is trained to jump toward an upright, white triangular figure in preference to an inverted white triangle, it will continue to react correctly in this choice when, for the first time, it is confronted with the mere outlines of these same figures in smaller size. Lashley comments that "here none of the retinal cells, and consequently none of the cells of the projection area which were stimulated by the contour of the figures during the training are similarly stimulated by the contours of the test figures." Lashley argues that this response of his test animals cannot depend upon the activation of any specific cells of the striate cortex, but rather upon a "pattern of excitation." In another series of experiments he trained rats to choose some simple figure, such as a circle, in preference to a square, and then destroyed portions of their striate cortex. He found that if the connecting pathways were left intact, he could destroy all but some six or seven hundred cortical cells, or 1/60th of the total, without abolishing the habitual response. As long as this minimum number of neurons remained functional, it apparently made no difference what portion of the striate cortex they might represent. On the other hand, if the rats were trained to respond to a more complex choice, requiring an element of judgment, almost any partial destruction of the striate cortex abolished the trained response.

As an example of this, with patience a rat can be trained to select from three circular figures, the middle sized one. Once that training period is complete, the rat will continue to make the proper choice with few mistakes, but now it is impossible to take away any considerable portion of his striate cortex without completely abolishing the trained response. These observations imply that for the rat trained to respond to the simple circle in preference to a square, a very few cells of the striate cortex were sufficient for the setting up of a pattern of excitation that was recognizable to the animal; but when the choice depended upon a more complicated problem, almost all, if not all, of the striate cortex was necessary for the establishment of a pattern of excitation that the rat could recognize.

The concept of "patterns of excitation" is not readily transposed into the commonly accepted interpretations of "neural transmission." The term implies the participation of many neuron units and, in the perception of complicated visual impressions, an activity of large areas of the sensory cortex functioning "as a whole." One is reminded of the cases with amnesia for the left side of the body which occurs in right-handed people, and which suggest an interaction of both cerebral hemispheres in the maintenance of a functionally integrated plastic model of self. Here again is the suggestion that large areas of the brain function as a whole. Other investigators of central nervous system function have touched on the same possibility, as when Coghill [12] talks of the "total pattern" of motor responses. But no one has been able to translate such a diffuse interaction into exact physiologic terminology. Lashley has not been able to express his concept of patterns of excitation in physiologic terms, but he utilizes an ingenious method for demonstrating what he means by the term. He puts the base of a vibrating tuning fork into a dish of mercury and makes a photograph or diagram of the concentric waves set up in the liquid mercury. Next he makes similar diagrams of the pool of mercury into which two tuning forks have been placed, then three, four, five, etc. A close inspection of the areas in which the waves, set up by more than one fork, overlap, will reveal that the pattern of reinforcement and interference is characteristic for each number of forks. If the observer is shown only a very small portion of the overlap area he may be able to identify the simple patterns, such as those set up by two, or possibly three forks. But to identify the more complex patterns, such as those set up by five or more forks, it is necessary that a much greater area be visualized in order that the pattern shall be recognizable.

I have an idea that the whole concept of "patterns of excitation" and the implication of large sensory centers functioning as an organic whole, will find increasing favor, even before its physiologic mechanisms are clarified. At least it seems to fit into the series of interpretations which I would like to reiterate in closing this chapter.

1. Pain is a perception, and as such is subject to the influence of associated ideas, apperceptions and fears.

2. The impulses which subserve it are not pain, but are merely a part of its underlying and alterable physical mechanisms.

3. The impulses may be initiated by a wide variety of stimuli; they are probably picked up by more than one type of receptor end-organ; certainly, they are carried by fibers of widely variant diameters and at quite different velocities.

4. When they enter the spinal cord they are subject to modi‚ fication by the internuncial pool of central neurons, whose activity is determined from moment to moment by other sensory impulses and by influences from other parts of the central nervous system.

5. In their ascent to the higher centers the impulses are subject to further modification at each functional level; the modifications at the various levels constituting an "integration" which fits them to subserve sensation.

6. In the sensorium they register as a "pattern of excitation" and from the resultant complex of sensory impressions, particular sensations, such as pain, may be recognized as the dominant feature.

SECTION TWO

# CLINICAL SYNDROMES

CHAPTER V

## Causalgia and Reflex Paralysis

"Causalgia" is a term now used to designate a clinical syndrome which may develop following a nerve injury. The syndrome occurs most frequently as a result of war wounds but is encountered occasionally in civil practice. The word itself means "burning pain" and was the term employed by Weir Mitchell to describe the pain that characterized some of his cases, and which he considered to be "the most terrible of all the tortures which a nerve wound may inflict." The condition is well illustrated by the following case which is quoted in full from Mitchell's book [85] (p. 292), "Nerve Injuries and Their Consequences."

CASE No. 47.—*Injury of median and ulnar nerves by a bullet; loss of motion; excessive causalgia; excision of four inches of median nerve; no relief.*

Jos. H. Corliss, late private Company B, 14th New York State Militia, aged twenty-seven, shingle-dresser, enlisted April, 1861, in good health. At the second battle of Bull Run August 29, 1862, he was shot in the left arm, three inches directly above the internal condyle. The ball emerged one and a quarter inches higher, through the belly of the biceps, without touching the artery, but with injury to the median and ulnar nerves. He was ramming a cartridge when hit and "thought he was struck on the crazy-bone by some of the boys for a 'joke.'" The fingers of both hands flexed and grasped the ramrod and gun tightly. Bringing the right hand, still clutching the ramrod, to the left elbow, he felt the blood and knew he was wounded. He then shook the ramrod from his grasp with a strong effort, and unloosened with the freed hand the tight grip of the left hand on the gun. After walking some twenty paces he fell from loss of blood, but still conscious; attempted to walk several times, and as often failed. He was finally helped to the rear, taken prisoner, lay three days on the field without food, but with enough of water to drink, and had his wounds dressed for the first time on the fourth day, at Fairfax Court House.

On the second day the pain began. It was burning and darting. He states that at this time sensation was lost or lessened in the limb, and that paralysis of motion came on in the hand and forearm. Admitted to the Douglas Hospital, Washington, D. C., September 7, 1862. The pain was so severe that a touch anywhere, or shaking the bed, or a heavy step, caused it to increase. The suffering was in the median and ulnar distribution, especially at the palmar face of the knuckles and the ball of the thumb. Motion has varied little since the wound, and as to sensation he is not clear.

Peter Pineo, surgeon, U. S. V., Medical Inspector, U. S. A., opened the wound and exsected two or three inches of the median nerve. The man states, very positively, that the pain in the median distribution did not cease, nor perceptibly lessen, but that he became more sensitive, so that even the rattling of a paper caused extreme suffering. He "thinks he was not himself" for a day or two after the operation. It seems quite certain that the pain afterwards gradually moderated, both in the ulnar and median tracts. Meanwhile the hand lay over his chest, and the fingers, flexing, became stiffened in this position.

About a week after he was shot, the *right* arm grew weak, and finally so feeble that he could not feed himself. He can now (April, 1864) use it pretty well, but it is manifestly less strong than the other. The left leg also was weakened, but when this loss of power first showed itself he cannot tell. He gives the usual account of the pain, and of the use of water on the hands and in his boots, as a means of easing it.

Present condition, April 21, 1864.—Wound healed. Cicatrix of the operation two and a half inches long over the median nerve. The forearm muscles do not seem to be greatly wasted. The interosseal muscles and hypothenar group are much atrophied, and the hand is thin and bony. The thenar muscles are partially wasted.

The skin of the palm is eczematous, thin, red and shining. The second and third phalanges of the fingers are flexed and stiff; the first is extended. Nails extraordinarily curved, laterally and longitudinally, except that of the thumb.

Pain is stated to exist still in the median distribution, but much less than in the ulnar tract, where it is excessively great.

He keeps his hand wrapped in a rag, wetted with cold water, and covered with oiled silk, and even tucks the rag carefully under the flexed finger tips. Moisture is more essential than cold. Friction outside of the clothes, at any point of the entire surface, "shoots" into the hand, increasing the burning in the median, sometimes, and more commonly, in the ulnar distribution. Deep pressure on the muscles has a like effect, and he will allow no one to touch his skin, save with a wetted hand, and even then is careful to exact careful manipulation. He keeps a bottle of water about him, and carries a sponge in the right hand. This hand he wets before he handles anything; used dry, it hurts the other limb. At one time, when the suffering was severe, he poured water into his boots, he says, to lessen the pain which dry touch or friction causes in the injured hand. So cautious was he about exposing the sore hand, that it was impossible thoroughly to examine it; but it was clear to us that there was sensibility in the ultimate median distribution, although he describes sensation as somewhat lessened in this region, and states that he has numbness on the inner side of the palm, and in the third and fourth fingers (ulnar tract). When the balls of the first and second fingers were touched, he said he felt it; but on touching those of the third and fourth fingers, he refused to permit us to experiment further, and insisted on wrapping up and wetting the hand. He thus describes the pain at its height. "It is as if a rough bar of iron were thrust to and fro through the knuckles, a red-hot iron placed at the junction of the palm and thenar eminence, with a heavy weight on it, and the skin was being rasped off my finger-ends."

In discussing causalgia, Mitchell [85] says (p. 196), "In our early experience of nerve wounds, we met with a small number of men who were suffering from a pain which they described as a 'burning,' or as a 'mustard red-hot,' or as a 'red-hot file rasping the skin.' In all of these patients, and in many later cases, this pain was an associate of the glossy skin previously described. In fact, this state of skin never existed without burning pain. Recently we have seen numbers of men who had burning pain without glossy skin, and in some we have seen this latter condition commencing. The burning comes first, the visible skin-change afterward; but in no case of great depravity in the nutrient condition of the skin have we failed to meet with it, and that in its forms of almost unendurable anguish. We have some doubts as to whether this form of pain ever originates at the moment of the wounding; but we have been so informed as regards two or three cases. Certain it is that, as a rule, the burning arises later, but almost always during the healing of the wound. Of the special cause which provokes it we know nothing, except that it has sometimes followed the transfer of pathologic changes from a wounded nerve to unwounded nerves, and has then been felt in their distribution, so that we do not need a direct wound to bring it about. The seat of the burning pain is very various; but it never attacks the trunk, rarely the arm or thigh, and not often the forearm or leg. Its favorite site is the foot or hand. In these parts it is to be found most often where the nutritive skin-changes are met with; that is to say, on the palm of the hand, or palmar face of the fingers, and on the dorsum of the foot; scarcely ever on the sole of the foot, or the back of the hand. When it first existed in the whole foot or hand, it always remained last in the parts above referred to, as its favorite seats. The great mass of sufferers described this pain as superficial, but others said it was also in the joints, and deep in the palm. If it lasted long it was finally referred to the skin alone."

It seems clear from these and other words of Mitchell's concerning "causalgia," that he had in mind the symptom of burning pain, and was not using the term to designate a definite clinical syndrome. However, in recent years this term has been used to designate a syndrome characterized by (1) *burning pain,* (2) extensive trophic changes, of which *glossy skin* is the most prominent, and (3) a local *rise in temperature,* in association with a wound of a peripheral nerve. Stopford [114] has suggested the term "thermalgia" for this syndrome, believing that the local rise in temperature is the most characteristic feature of the symptom-complex.

In some respects it is unfortunate that "causalgia" should be reserved for this combination of signs and symptoms, particularly when the emphasis is placed on the presence of a local hyperthermia, because the complete combination of features is exceedingly rare. In relatively few instances of what I would call causalgia, is a local rise in temperature seen as a persistent feature. More often, when it does occur, it is transient and is followed by a fall in temperature so that the involved part is colder than normal. In my experience only two cases come to mind that could be called "typical causalgia" if the co-existence of all three features is considered essential to such a diagnosis. On the other hand, cases with burning pain and cases with glossy skin, or these two in association with one another, occur with such frequency as to suggest that they are among the common sequelae of nerve irritation. In a study of a large group of peripheral nerve lesions, Pollock and Davis[98] noted the presence of "glossy skin" in forty-one cases in which burning pain was not an associated finding; and of thirty-eight cases characterized by burning pain, only eight showed glossy skin. They do not mention the relationship of local hyperthermia in connection with these findings, but it is apparent that the number of their cases which would show all three features must have been very small.

It is my opinion that the three features are separate manifestations of nerve irritation, which only in rare instances occur in combination. There are other trophic changes in addition to that of glossy skin that could be emphasized, coldness is undoubtedly more frequently found than local heat, and hyperesthesia and sweating certainly deserve prominent places in any consideration of the manifestations of irritative lesions of sensory nerves. All of these features will be found to occur in quite variable combinations, so much so that it is a misleading and artificial distinction to select three of them and designate them as a clinical entity. It would have been better perhaps if the term "causalgia" had been restricted as Mitchell employed it, i.e., to describe the single symptom of burning pain. Since, however, it is now customary to use it to designate a clinical syndrome, I shall use it, but in a broad sense, as applicable to the severe case of nerve irritation in which burning pain is a prominent feature. For the less severe type of case of nerve irritation I shall employ the term "minor causalgia" as suggested by Homans.[54] A third group of cases will be reported under the title "post-traumatic pain syndromes." I do not like this designation, but as these patients do not complain of burning pain, it does not seem logical to designate them as causalgias. It should be understood that such classifications are not, in my opinion, significant of essential distinctions. To me they are all manifestations of sensory nerve irritation and probably they all have a similar underlying *pathologic physiology*.*

As to the duration of causalgia, Mitchell leaves the impression that the burning pain and the other signs and symptoms of nerve irritation tend to be self-limited, and after a period of months, or at least a year or two, gradually disappear. Pollock and Davis [98] write that "the condition reaches its height four or five months after injury and tends to disappear slowly. Many cases so continue for a period of two years." Such a view might well encourage the physician to adopt a "watchful-waiting" policy. I feel strongly that the waiting policy can be, and usually is, overdone. There are two principal reasons for this opinion. In the first place, there is no limit to the time that the symptoms may persist. Mitchell [85] comments on a case that was cured of causalgia after sixteen years of pain; and when, in 1895, John Mitchell [82] reviewed the subsequent histories of some of the cases his father had written about thirty years earlier, it was surprising how many of them had suffered pain and disability for long periods after they left Turner's Lane hospital. Leriche [64] mentions a case, "who, seventeen years after his wound, was suffering from his causalgia more than ever." He says further: "It is true that, left to itself, the causalgia may sometimes undergo a process of gradual cure. But there are a number of cases which have been followed up for a long time, and which demonstrate that, sometimes, far from clearing up, the condition may become steadily worse and worse; the area of distribution of the pain extending, and the manifestations of vasomotor disorder continuing to spread."

* The terms "pathologic physiology" and "abnormal physiology" involve an obvious contradiction; nevertheless they have been used here to imply a disturbance in physiologic processes in contrast to organic change in anatomic structure.

A second reason for not adopting a waiting policy is perhaps the more important one. The damage that may be done during even a relatively short waiting period may be irretrievable. Not only may the skin become thin, red, glossy and devoid of wrinkles; but the muscles may undergo fibrous changes so that they become almost immovable; and the bones show atrophy, which may vary from a slight generalized loss of density, to the spongy, "moth-eaten" appearance of an advanced osteoporosis. The skin no longer slides easily over the underlying structures but fuses with them, the small joints are stiffened and fixed, and the fingers become thin and tapering. The pain and hyperesthesia are so great that the patient will not submit to massage or manipulations which might improve tissue nutrition and maintain mobility of muscles and joints. Heat usually seems to aggravate the pain, so that the usual modalities of physiotherapy are, for all practical purposes, excluded. In many instances, by the time something is done to alleviate the pain, the tissue damage is so extensive and far advanced that no amount of treatment will now restore normal function. And the alterations in "morale," emotional stability, and even in personality, which may result from long-continued suffering, are not the least important of the permanent changes which may be left, even when the burden of pain can be lifted.

The treatment of causalgia is frequently difficult and the results unsatisfactory, particularly when the treatment is instituted late, if the spreading signs and symptoms are severe and have been present a long time. When the irritative lesion involves a major nerve, and when the evidences of this irritation show no tendency to subside, but instead get steadily worse, the nerve should at once be exposed surgically. If it is apparent that the damage is not serious, a neurolysis should be carried out, and, if possible, the trunk placed in a new bed at a distance from the scar tissue resulting from the original injury. If the nerve has been partially divided, an excision of the damaged portion and an immediate end-to-end suture of the divided trunk, may effect a cure. Occasionally, a cure has been reported from an excision of appropriate sympathetic ganglia, without anything being done to the original nerve lesion. The reason why such a procedure may be successful will require more discussion in subsequent chapters.

But these methods, or any combination of them may fail, as is evident in the following case summary.

CASE No. 5.—Mr. C. S., a 35-year-old worker in a lumber mill, was struck by a flying belt on November 25, 1935, and thrown against a timber. The upper third of the right humerus was fractured transversely. From the time of the accident, he complained bitterly of pain. There was an aching pain in the upper arm and a burning pain in the hand. The ring and little fingers felt "numb" and "half asleep," subjectively, but at the same time were extremely sensitive to the lightest touch. Several times each day the forearm muscles would go into a cramp so that the fingers, particularly the ring and little fingers, would be drawn tightly into the palm and the patient "had to work them loose with the other hand." It was noted that these two fingers sweated excessively and were constantly discolored and cold.

I examined this man for the first time more than two years after his injury. He kept the hand carefully guarded from any contact and was reluctant to have it examined. The ring and little fingers, particularly the distal two joints of the ring finger, were red and shiny and the nails were opaque and long. He dared not cut these two nails because it so aggravated his pain, but at times they were accidentally broken off. The ulnar side of the hand was glistening wet with perspiration and when he hung the hand down the drops of sweat dripped from the end of the ring finger every few seconds. In spite of the subjective sensation of burning in the hand, it was colder than the left hand; the ring and little fingers measuring 2° C. colder than the same fingers of the left hand. The fractured humerus had never united. During the two years since his accident four operations had been carried out on the arm in an effort to secure bony union. The first "sliding-graft" had absorbed soon after it was put in place. Twice the Boehler procedure of boring holes in the callus ends had been tried, and then a large graft was taken from his tibia, but this, too, had disappeared. There was some fibrous union present, but movement at the fracture site or any pressure on the arm in this region aggravated his pains to an intolerable degree. The man looked thin and pain-worn and had lost 22 pounds since his accident. He stated: "My whole right side seems to be affected; my right eye blurs when I try to read; my chest and neck on that side hurt most of the time and my right leg is weak and often gives way under me."

Examination of the arm showed an enlargement of the ulnar nerve trunk at the level of the ununited fracture. A small amount of novocaine solution injected into the trunk above this lump gave him relief from pain for several hours. There were two other methods by which temporary relief could be conferred. One was to inject the upper thoracic sympathetic ganglia (2nd, 3rd and 4th) with novocaine. The other was a similar injection of the ulnar nerve at the elbow. This last is of interest because the injection was several inches *distal* to the irritative lesion. On May 18, 1938, the nerve was exposed in the upper arm and found to be partially divided and the protruding lateral mass of fibers imbedded in a highly vascular scar tissue. This segment of the nerve was excised and an end-to-end suture carried out. There was, of course, the usual change in the hand that follows an interruption of the ulnar nerve. But the relief from pain was complete and the change in the patient himself was dramatic. But after two months some of the pain began to recur and by October it was as bad as ever.

Between November, 1938, and April, 1939, a series of novocaine injections were carried out, blocking successively the ulnar nerve above the anastomosis, the brachial plexus, and the stellate ganglion. A second resection of the nerve and a new anastomosis not only failed to confer relief, but seemed to aggravate the whole pain picture. Thereafter a combination of injections of the stellate ganglion and of the anastomotic area were sufficient to hold his pain under reasonable control until early in 1940. Then the effectiveness of these injections seemed to diminish and a stellate block on February 13, 1940, was said to aggravate his pain. In July, 1940, a third resection of the nerve was done, and this time he again experienced complete relief. In September he reportd a gain of twelve pounds in weight and was sleeping and eating well. There was less local sensitiveness in the operative area than at any time previously. He remained quite comfortable until the middle of October, when he caught a cold, and hard coughing spells brought back the pain in the chest, axilla and upper arm and within a few weeks his pain was again as bad as ever, with the entire right side affected. At his request the nerve was exposed again, and this time permanently sacrificed, the cut end being buried in the deltoid muscle well away from the scar tissue area. The relief conferred by the operation was only partial and in the next few months the pain gradually returned to its full force.

Before resorting to a high chordotomy or a resection of the posterior roots of the brachial plexus, two more attempts were made to secure bony union at the fracture site, acting on the theory that irritation caused by slight movement there might be keeping active the pain process. The first attempt failed because he simply could not tolerate his cast. The second attempt, carried out late in 1941, resulted in a solid union and since then there has been a progressive diminution on all of his complaints.

This is a tragic case. It might be said, with a certain justification, that this patient was over-treated, and that left alone he would have fared better. I doubt it. Nor do I believe that to have secured a solid union of the fracture, without doing anything to the injured nerve, would have proven sufficient in this case. I have the conviction, not without some clinical basis, that if the nerve lesion had been resected in the first few months of his suffering, that procedure alone would have solved the pain problem, whether or not anything had been done then to assure a bony union. Looking back now, it seems likely that even at the late date the first resection was carried out, this operation might have proven permanently successful in relieving the pain if, at the same time, the "step operation" on the fractured humerus had been successfully accomplished. However, I am not relating this case because of any lesson to be learned from the treatment. Nor is this the place to give my own interpretations of the pain mechanisms acting in this case of ulnar causalgia. The case serves well to illustrate the harm that can result from a single irritative nerve lesion and the spreading nature of its symptomatology.

### REFLEX PARALYSIS

The second important contribution in the field of neurology that was made by Weir Mitchell and his associates, Morehouse and Keen, was a paper dealing with "Reflex Paralysis." [84] A circular under this title was issued from the Surgeon General's office in March, 1864, "For the information of Medical Officers, in the belief that immediate and practical benefit may be derived from it."

This paper contains much of interest aside from its principal topic. These men recognized primary and secondary shock and described cases of collapse from proximity to an explosion without signs of external injury, a condition which is recognized in the present war under the term "primary blast." In commenting on shock, this was said: "The majority of physicians will no doubt be disposed to attribute the chief share in the phenomena of shock in its various forms, to the indirect influence exerted upon and through the heart. There are, however, certain facts, which duly considered, will, we think, lead us to suppose that in many cases the phenomena in question may be due to a temporary paralysis of the whole range of nerve centres, and that among these phenomena the cardiac feebleness may play a large part, and be itself induced by the state of the regulating nerve centres of the great circulatory organ."

Of equal interest are the comments on "commotion" in nerves and nerve centers brought about by mechanical agencies, such as the violent jarring of the tissues by bullets in close proximity to parts of the central nervous system structures. To quote again: "If, for example, a ball passes near the spinal column, it is conceivable that the roll of its motion, and the resistance of the tissues, may determine in the spine a brusque and sudden oscillation of the contents, sufficient to cause very grave results." The importance of this view is indicated in the present-day investigation of head injuries. For instance, it is found that a blow of sufficient force to shatter the skull may be delivered against the head of an experimental animal, and so long as the head is held firm, as in a vice or against an immovable support, the animal will survive. But if a blow of exactly the same force is delivered against the unfixed and freely movable head, the animal is killed. This observation is quite the opposite to what might have been anticipated, but the experimental findings are apparently dependent upon the fact that with the head movable, the blow creates the "sudden oscillation of the contents," and with the same "grave results" that Mitchell commented on more than three-quarters of a century ago.

But the authors make a distinction between nerve "commotion" and shock, and the condition which they term "Reflex Paralysis." They write: "We have seen that in all probability the state of shock from gun shot injuries is a state of general paralysis. We have also seen that in the great mass of cases it is temporary. We have now to show that in rare instances the paralysis continues as a more or less permanent evil, after the general depression has passed away. When, therefore, a wound occurs, and the patient surviving the first effect is found to have paralysis of a distant limb or limbs, it is impossible to deny to such cases the title of reflex paralysis. All of the following instances seem to us to have fulfilled every condition which would entitle them to be so considered."

Then follows a most interesting series of seven case histories, in each one of which there was a "paralysis of a remote part or parts occasioned by a gun-shot wound of some prominent nerve, or of some part of the body which is richly supplied with nerve branches of secondary size and importance." In one, the wound involved the muscles of the neck or throat and the hyoid bone, and it was followed by a paralysis of both arms. The effects of this paralysis soon disappeared in the left arm except for a slight residual diminution of tactile sensibility in the distribution of the ulnar nerve, but the right arm remained greatly enfeebled and the source of constant pain for many months. In another case, a wound of the thigh muscles external to the femoral artery on the right side, was followed not only by a persisting paralysis of the injured leg, but also of the right arm and the left leg. To a remarkable degree the involvement of the left leg "reflected" that seen in the leg of the injured side. In a third case, a musket-ball passed obliquely through the right thigh, and was followed by paralysis of the right leg and arm. The paralysis of the leg was attributed to "commotion" in the sciatic nerve which lay close to the track of the ball, but the arm paralysis was considered to be "reflex."

The details of these seven case histories are worthy of study, but no purpose is served by relating them all here. However, the authors' comments on these cases are of sufficient significance in relation to the central theme of this monograph to be quoted more freely. "In three of these cases the leg was hit, and the arm of the same side was paralyzed. In three cases the paralysis affected the opposite side of the body, and in one the paralysis of tact and pain was observed to have fallen upon a space symmetrically related to the wounded spot as regards position. No general law, therefore, can be deduced from these records, nor from what we see in the causation of reflex paralysis from disease should we expect any inevitable relation between the part injured and the consequent paralysis. The constitutional condition at the time of the wounding, as to excitement, mental and physical, may possibly have to do with causing the resultant paralysis. . . . The after-history of these cases is extremely curious. However grave the lesion of motion or sensation, it grew better early in the case, and continued to improve until the part had nearly recovered all its normal powers. In almost every instance some relic of the paralysis remained, even after eighteen months or more from the date of wounding. In some, the part remained weak; in others, there was still left some slight loss of sensibility, and in two the loss of power and sensory appreciation was very considerable. In a case of reflex paralysis from a wound we have, therefore, some right to expect that the patient will recover rapidly up to a certain point; then in most cases a small amount of loss of power or sensation may remain."

In discussing the possible causes for the reflex paralysis, the authors consider various mechanisms which might explain their observations. They are inclined to reject the theory that the wound brings about any long-sustained capillary contraction in the nerve centers. They consider it more likely that any primary constriction of the capillary bed would be transient, perhaps to be followed by a relaxation of these vessels to an extent that might constitute a "congestion." They point out, if nutritive changes occurred, on the basis of either capillary constriction or dilatation, there should be evidences in the nerve centers which the pathologist should be able to demonstrate. In the absence of such confirmatory evidence they are inclined to favor the view that severe injuries may be competent to exhaust the irritability of nerve centers, so as to produce a loss of function, which might prove more or less permanent.

"It appears to us possible that a very severe injury of a part may be competent to so exhaust the irritability of the nerve centres, as to give rise to loss of function, which might prove more or less permanent. A strong electric current, frequently interrupted, is certainly able to cause such a result in a nerve trunk, while in general electric shock, as a stroke of lightning, is, as we well know, quite competent to destroy the irritability of every excitable tissue in the economy. Now if the former of these results can occur in a nerve so insulated as practically to have no circulation, the loss of irritability cannot be set down in such a case to a defect of circulation. Reflecting then upon the close correlation of the electrical and neural force, it does not seem improbable that a violent excitement of a nerve trunk should be able to exhaust completely the power of its connected nerve centre."

The writings of these authors on causalgia and reflex paralysis have much more than an historical importance. Nor have I devoted space to this brief summary merely to call attention to the acumen these men exhibited in their observations and interpretations. Both causalgia and reflex paralysis have assumed a new importance in the present world conflict, and instead of being called upon to treat the occasional, isolated case from civilian practice, surgeons all over the world will be suddenly faced with the urgent necessity for recognizing and treating both of these conditions. They will be confronted by cases that exhibit sensory changes and the loss of motor function so bizarre in their distribution, and apparently so unrelated to the apparent causes as to throw doubt on there being any possible organic basis for them. They will be called upon to treat syndromes which may be "the most terrible of all the tortures which a nerve wound may inflict." They will observe functional and trophic disturbances of wide distribution that may not conform to any pattern of nerve distribution which their textbooks had taught them to expect. Because of these things there will be a great temptation to deny to such cases an organic basis, and to ascribe the symptoms to psychic causes for which the patient may in some way be responsible.

I am not concerned primarily with this possibility as it relates to the clear-cut cases of either causalgia or reflex paralysis. They occur in the texts dealing with nerve injuries. And in the cases with pain of such degree as to strain the observer's credulity, the pain will doubtless be associated with so many physical signs of functional and trophic change as to make the organic nature of the syndrome apparent and the diagnosis obvious.

My concern is for the infinitely greater number of wounded soldiers and civilian casualties whose complaints may have an equally real organic basis, but whose physical signs are not of sufficient degree to make this fact apparent. It is this group that is in danger of being misunderstood and discredited. They are the ones who are in danger of mismanagement or neglect for sufficiently long periods as to permit the underlying pathologic physiology to secure a complete ascendency over normal function.

## CHAPTER VI

## Minor Causalgia

For several years it was a part of my job as Medical Examiner for the Oregon State Industrial Accident Commission to examine injured workmen whose cases presented specific problems relating to treatment or disability rating. Among these cases there were a considerable number of finger amputations. The symptoms elicited from the men who were most dissatisfied with the prescribed "permanent partial disability ratings" based on purely anatomic considerations, were almost always the same. Over and over I heard this combination of complaints: "The stump pains all the time; it is always cold; and I can hardly bear to let anything touch it." The superficial hyperesthesia was readily demonstrable, and in many cases the impairment of circulation was equally obvious. The stump and often the whole hand might be colder and more cyanotic than the normal hand, and exposure to cold brought out the difference even more clearly. The pain was most commonly described as an ache, sometimes as a "burning" and it became worse when the hand was cold or when exposed to heat. In the worst of these cases the combination of burning pain, vasomotor and sudomotor disturbances and the dusky-red, shiny and smooth, thin skin of the stump and neighboring parts, was strongly suggestive of the principal features of causalgia.

There is, of course, in these cases no lesion of a large nerve trunk, and they have no such widespread and dramatic functional and structural changes as was seen in the classical syndrome of causalgia. But it might be permissible, as Homans [54] has done, to classify cases of this type as "minor causalgia." One can find a whole series of cases having these same characteristics, that vary in severity and importance all the way from the simple finger amputation to the case of Joseph Corliss, which has been quoted from Mitchell's text in the preceding chapter. I believe that each one of such a series is dependent upon the chronic irritation of sensory nerve fibers, and that the characteristic features are reflex in origin and are dependent upon a disturbed central physiology. Just why one particular finger amputation is followed by the development of a profound physiologic disturbance, while the great majority of similar injuries show only minor changes for a short period of time, or are spared entirely, no one is able to say. The psychic make-up of the patient may have something to do with it. It may be that, as Leriche [65] has suggested, "causalgia is a disease which must be regarded as a function of the temperament of the individual." But I cannot subscribe wholly to this view. It is quite possible that persons of a particular temperament are more prone to develop it than others, but I have seen cases with both hands injured at the same time, and each similarly involved, in which one side heals "normally" and the other develops the syndrome suggestive of causalgia. I suspect that the underlying cause is more directly related to the manner in which sensory nerves become involved in scar or are otherwise subjected to a chronic irritation.

The cases which will be considered in this and the subsequent chapter differ from one another in many respects, but in them all will be found evidences of a similar disturbed physiology. As regards their physical aspects they constitute a very heterogeneous group. DeTakats [18] has discussed cases of this general type under the term "reflex dystrophy"; Leriche [65] includes similar cases under the title, "post-traumatic spreading neuralgia"; Flothow [26] has termed them "sympathalgia"; I have reported some under two titles, as "post-traumatic pain syndromes" and as "irritative nerve lesions"; [74] and Homans [54] tends to call them all, "minor causalgias." It is quite probable that as our knowledge of this general group increases, we will learn to make distinctions between significant subgroups. For the present it is not so important what we call them, as long as it is understood what we mean by the term. I shall describe different aspects of the same group of cases in two chapters, the present one under the title, "minor causalgia," and the next one under "post-traumatic pain syndromes." I include under the first term all those cases, of lesser degree than the classical instance of "major causalgia," in which burning pain was a feature of the syndrome. Under "post-traumatic pain syndromes" I include the remainder of the group in which burning pain is not an obvious feature of the complaints. The reader should bear in mind that I consider the distinctions between the two groups to be artificial, and that whether or not burning pain figures in the pain picture, the underlying pathologic physiology is the same.

In spite of individual differences between the cases of this heterogeneous group of "irritative nerve lesion" cases, the clinical picture for the group as a whole possesses several unusual features. In the first place, the pain and the physical signs may not conform to the known patterns of distribution of the peripheral nerves or of the nerve roots. In the second place, a local hyperesthesia is very common. When this hyperesthesia is excessive and it occurs without any striking evidence of organic pathology, the observer is prone to underestimate its severity or doubt its reality. A third unusual feature is the frequent association of physical signs indicating an abnormal activity of nerve function, particularly of the sympathetic nerves. Among these are local sweating, alterations in color and temperature, local edema, and "trophic" changes involving the skin, muscles, joints and bones. The trophic changes develop insidiously and when well advanced they may be irreversible, so that the functional efficiency of the limb may be permanently impaired. Trophic changes are baffling to the surgeon because they are so difficult to cure, and to the physiologist because they cannot be readily reproduced in the experimental animal, nor can they be easily explained.

The most unusual feature of these cases is their tendency to improve when the local area of injury or the appropriate sympathetic ganglia are infiltrated with novocaine solution. There is no good evidence that this drug destroys the nerve pathways that are so injected, and normal sensation usually returns to the part promptly and completely. Yet many clinical observers have reported instances in which a single injection of novocaine has permanently abolished, not only this type of pain syndrome, but the syndrome of trigeminal neuralgia, angina pectoris, dysmenorrhea, etc. Sometimes the dramatic character of the cure partakes of the supernatural. It cannot be doubted that such cures occur, but if the fact is accepted, the cure is attributed to a form of suggestion therapy, having as its motivating forces a desire to get well, a surgical procedure that affords immediate relief, combined with, perhaps, the persuasive influence of the surgeon himself.

This combination of unusual features influences many observers to believe that these cases have no organic basis. Even the physical signs of vasomotor disturbance and tissue change might be explained as secondary to influences from the hypothalamus which are activated by the same thalamic and cerebral perturbations to which the exaggerated pain responses could be ascribed. But these cases are no less real than those we recognize under the names, "Sudeck's atrophy," "meralgia paresthetica," "scalenus anticus syndrome," "traumatic osteoporosis," "Volkmann's ischemic paralysis," etc. In fact, it is very probable that all of these well-recognized clinical states are related to those under discussion and depend upon a similar reflex dystrophy.

The treatment recommended for these cases is varied. Some of them tend to get well spontaneously, and those that are not too sensitive to permit the use of physiotherapy, seem to improve more rapidly under the use of heat, massage and active use of the part. Many of them cannot tolerate these agencies, and left to themselves, tend to get progressively worse. Sometimes, if a particularly tender part is first injected with novocaine, the sensitiveness of the whole hand or foot is sufficiently reduced to permit massage and active exercise during the period the anesthetic effect persists. Where the symptoms develop following a partial amputation of a digit, a higher amputation may stop the process, but as often as not this method fails. Leriche [64] has recommended periarterial sympathectomy for this syndrome and reports many successful results. I have carried out this form of "sympathectomy" but few times, and am unable to evaluate the method. I certainly agree with Leriche that if an artery is sufficiently injured to obliterate its lumen, the obliterated segment should be excised. I am convinced that the arteries are richly supplied with sensory fibers, and that their nerves, if subjected to chronic irritation, are almost as prone as are other sensory nerves, to set up a disturbed local physiology. But I have been inclined, when I think a sympathectomy is indicated, to attack the sympathetic ganglia rather than carry out a periarterial stripping. However, Homans [54] has recently reported some cases that have been benefited by

· this relatively simple procedure, and it is quite possible that when the rationale of the operation is better understood, it may enjoy a wider favor than at present.

A sympathetic ganglionectomy has "cured" many of these cases, and some surgeons are inclined to resort to such an operation as a method of first choice. When the syndrome involves a lower extremity, it is quite generally agreed that it is best to excise the second and third lumbar sympathetic ganglia and sometimes the first ganglion as well. For conditions involving the upper extremity the focus of the surgical attack is less definitely agreed upon. But since, in the syndromes under discussion, the permanency of the sympathetic interruption is perhaps of less concern than in cases such as Raynaud's disease, it seems that any procedure which interrupts the vasomotor nerves to the part has a good chance of being successful. This problem will come up for further comment in the chapter, "The Sympathetic Component."

When the location of the offending lesion can be identified, the simplest method of treatment consists in an excision of the area. When the excision is carried out early, relief seems to be conferred more often than when it is done late. But before local excision or any attack on the sympathetic nerves is undertaken it is well worth while trying repeated novocaine injections of the offending site of trouble. Many of my cases have responded favorably to this method alone. In the successful cases the hyperesthesia disappears and coincidentally the pain is relieved; not only the local pain, but also pain felt at a considerable distance away in the distribution of other nerves than that supplying the part being injected. Not infrequently, too, there is a remarkable increase in the mobility of joints and in muscle strength following the injection. With these changes there may be an accompanying improvement in the local circulation, as evidenced by warming and an improvement in the color of the part. These signs of improvement may last only a few hours, to be followed by a recurrence of the pain syndrome in its original severity, or perhaps even temporarily aggravated. The syndrome does not *always* recur as soon as the local anesthetic effect of the drug has worn off. Quite often the relief persists for days, weeks, or months, and sometimes it is permanent. And of the considerable percentage of cases in which the relief following one injection proves to be temporary, an encouraging number may be "cured" by repeated injections.

CASE No. 6.—*Minor Causalgia. Treated by Excision of Trigger Point.*

Mrs. M. P., a housewife of 61, was referred on May 21, 1937, for pain and disability involving the right arm and hand. In January, 1936, she suffered from an attack of herpes zoster for which her physician had given her an intravenous injection. The solution (probably sodium iodide) was injected in or around a vein on the lateral aspect of the right cubital fossa. She complained of severe pain during and after this injection. The arm swelled markedly and required treatment by hot packs and the support of a sling for five weeks. During this time the pain was said to be intense, preventing sleep and necessitating repeated hypodermic injections of morphine sulphate. A hard mass, about the size of an egg, was left as the generalized swelling subsided. It remained sensitive to pressure. The fingers of the right hand became stiff, the skin assumed a reddish color and appeared thin and glossy. She described two types of pain —one, a constant burning "as if the hand were too hot," and the other a tingling, prickling sensation "as if the hand had been asleep." The pains were most severe on the ulnar side of the forearm and hand, the cubital fossa and the posterior aspect of the shoulder. Use aggravated the pain. She could not hold objects securely in the right hand, and was unable to write well, and the outer side of the forearm became so hyperesthetic that she could not rest it on a table.

Touching the lump near the elbow caused "electric shocks" to run down the forearm and "out" through the ends of the fingers. She had received a variety of treatments with no benefit. Diathermy could not be tolerated.

Examination showed the right hand to be mottled and red but there was no excessive sweating. Thermocouple readings of skin temperature showed the fingers to be about 1° C. colder than those of the left hand. The skin was thin and glistening and seemed to be fused with the atrophic deeper tissues. The fifth finger was completely stiff except for about ten degrees of flexion at the metacarpophalangeal joint. The ring finger could be flexed about halfway to the palm, and the mid-finger about three-quarters of that distance. The thumb was said to "feel more stiff" than it actually was to passive motion. The index finger had a normal range of motion and was less involved in the color changes and subjective complaints than was the remainder of the hand. Both wrist arteries pulsated well. She complained of tenderness when the right brachial vessels were compressed. On the lateral aspect of the cubital fossa were two hard masses, very close together and fixed to the underlying tissues and the skin. They were about the size of hazelnuts and were only slightly tender to direct pressure. However, when they were pressed upon she complained of a tingling shock that was transmitted down into the fingers.

On June 2, 1937, the local masses were excised under local anesthesia. A wide diffusion of the procaine solution was necessary to secure adequate anesthesia. The masses were difficult to remove because the scar extended much more widely than palpation seemed to indicate, and there was much oozing from tiny vessels. Histological examination of the tissue removed showed it to be dense scar tissue in which could be recognized a segment of a vein.

The patient was certain that the operation had conferred benefit within 24 hours, and by the time the skin sutures were removed she had less stiffness and more strength in the hand, and the color and temperature of the fingers were equal in the two hands. Three months after the operation she wrote stating that she had excellent use of the hand, had lost much of her "nervousness," and all of her pain and hyperesthesia, and considered herself "cured."

In November, 1937, she reported that the scar was becoming sensitive, but the threat of a recurrence proved transient, and when she was last examined in July, 1941, she stated that she was completely free from symptoms. The function of her hand was normal.

CASE No. 7.—*Minor Causalgia. Treated by Novocaine Blockade of Sensory Nerves.*

Mrs. H. B., aged 76, was referred for examination on March 9, 1937, complaining of "terrible" pain in the right hand. In August, 1936, she had had a cholecystectomy performed, and for several days, while critically ill, had had many intravenous injections of normal saline and glucose. About a month after she left the hospital she began to have attacks of sharp, tingling pain in the right hand and fingers that would waken her each night. Between the sharp attacks of pain there was a constant sensation as of "electricity going through the tips of the fingers." The thumb, index and middle fingers were constantly involved in the sensation, the ring finger, occasionally, but the little finger, never. When this sensation was severe it ascended the hand to the wrist or the elbow. With the sharper burning pains was associated a burning feeling, "as if all of a sudden I got it on fire." If at such times she put her fingers against her face she found that they were warmer than the fingers of the other hand. Heat definitely aggravated the pain, an ice bag did not relieve it, but mild cooling sometimes afforded slight benefit. Walking around seemed to ease the pain, and she said she had spent most of her nights walking the floor. Rubbing the hand did not diminish the pain. There was a slight swelling of the hand, more marked when she first got up in the morning than later. It was hard for her to make a fist. Writing and sewing had become very difficult. She claimed to be exhausted from lack of sleep and insisted that the pain she had suffered after her gall-bladder operation could not compare with one night of pain in her hand.

There was no definite swelling or discoloration of the hand at the time of the first examination and the fingers were about 2° C. colder on the affected side. Because the distribution of the pain suggested an involvement of the median nerve, this nerve was selected for block. The novocaine was injected just above the elbow level and within a few minutes the index and middle finger tips warmed 4° C., and there was a slight subjective sense of numbness in the index finger but no complete anesthesia. She reported on March 15 that she had had one very comfortable day and night immediately following the injection, and for the remainder of the week had been up during the night much less than usual. The same injection was repeated and four days later she reported that the benefit was brief. The ulnar nerve was then injected, but this procedure produced no change whatever in her complaints. Six more injections of the median nerve were carried out at increasing intervals up to May 28, 1937. On this date she stated that her pains had become steadily less frequent and severe and that she had not been awakened at night for some time. There was an occasional sensation of burning heat in the fingers, but it was mild in degree and the tingling sensations had entirely disappeared. Examined on August 3 there was no measurable difference in the temperature of the fingers of the two hands, no burning sensation, no tingling and no swelling. She could hold a needle, write as well as before the onset of her trouble. She considered herself well, but said she would report for further injections if her symptoms recurred. She last reported on January 15, 1938, as needing no more treatment and considered herself "completely cured."

CASE No. 8.—*Intermittent Minor Causalgia. Treated by Local Infiltration.*

Mrs. G. E. A., aged 58, was referred for treatment of periodic pain in her right foot on September 9, 1937. Three years previously she fell and injured this foot. The outer side of the foot at the base of the toes turned "black and blue," but x-ray plates did not reveal any fractures. As the ecchymosis cleared she noted that the outer three toes "felt dead." Later she began to have periodic pains "like a toothache" in these toes and during such attacks all three would be extremely sensitive to touch. The attacks continued with increasing frequency and severity, sometimes occurring several times a day, and occasionally skipping a day or two, but never longer. There was no true anesthesia, but the threshold for light touch was raised. The subjective feeling of "deadness" seemed to increase just before an attack began—next she experienced a sensation of swelling in the toes beginning at their bases on the plantar surface and spreading to involve all three toes to their junction with the foot. At its height she said the toes felt "as if bursting and on fire." During the attack she was unable to tolerate the lightest touch to the toes. She had never noted any change in color, temperature or sweating of these toes even during an attack. For the previous two years the outer three toes of the other foot had felt "slightly numb and dead" and on several occasions she had experienced twinges of pain in them which made her fear that "the trouble is going over into the other foot."

Nothing of significance was found in physical examination. She received ten injections of a 2 per cent novocaine solution into the dorsum of the foot at the base of the toes. Each injection was followed by a period of complete relief from attacks, and these intervals of freedom became increasingly long as the treatment progressed. The last injection was given on March 18, 1938, since which time there has been no recurrence of pain.

To the attending physician the majority of cases of minor causalgia are annoying and trying. The onset of symptoms may follow the most commonplace of injuries. A bruise, a superficial cut, the prick of a thorn or a broken chicken-bone, a sprain or even a postoperative scar may act as the causative lesion. The event which precipitates the syndrome may appear both to the patient and the physician as of minor consequence, and both have every reason to anticipate the same prompt recovery that follows similar injuries. This anticipation is not realized and the symptoms tend to become progressively worse. Physiotherapy may increase the burning pain and is therefore resisted by the patient. His resistance and the inexplicable persistence of his complaints may lead to an alienation of the physician's sympathy. It may seem that the patient doesn't want to cooperate or that he has some ulterior motive in resisting the efforts to improve his condition. Sometimes these explanations are true, but in most instances I believe that the resistance is prompted by the aggravation of the burning pain that treatment entails.

It is here that novocaine injection may be of assistance because a preliminary infiltration of the sensitive scar or a deep trigger point may make it possible for heat treatments and massage to be carried out during the short period that the region is anesthetic. In addition, the expanding effect exerted on the sensitive scar tissues by the injection seems to have a favorable effect, perhaps by relieving compression of sensory nerve filaments. As an example of what I have in mind, let me cite the example of a mill worker who lost the distal half of his right thumb in a crushing accident. Examination eight months after the accident revealed that there was an extreme degree of hyperesthesia, coldness and wasting of the thumb muscles. The index finger, which had not been involved in the accident, was also obviously wasted, the pad of this fingertip being lax, wrinkled and thin. The man complained bitterly of burning pain and was deeply incensed at his attending physician because "everything he does to me makes me worse." A reamputation of the remaining portion of the distal phalanx had not lessened the complaints; in fact, had seemingly made them worse. The man complained that heat treatments were simply "intolerable" and the lightest attempts at massage "a torture."

He was also aggrieved because the State Accident Commission had twice closed his case with what seemed to him an insignificant disability award. He was determined that he would "make them pay and pay well." His attitude was distinctly prejudicial to his own interests, but the condition of the affected digit left no doubt that his disability was real. The scar tissue over the end of the stump was dense and adherent to the underlying bone. In order to infiltrate novocaine into this dense scar it was necessary to begin the injection well down toward the base of the thumb and progress upward. The injection was unquestionably most painful as the tense tissues were being distended. As soon as the injection was complete, however, both heat and vigorous massage could be used. Four such treatments were sufficient to loosen up the scar tissue and lessen the sensitiveness to a degree that permitted further treatment without any preliminary injection of local anesthetic. Within a month this workman was free from symptoms and back on the job.

In interpreting the factors that led to improvement in this case, it is difficult to decide which of the various procedures was chiefly responsible for the cure. The same question arises in the treatment of any sensitive scar that can be similarly treated. Does the local anesthetic deserve the chief credit, or is the expansion of the dense scar the major factor, or is it the physiotherapy that must be credited with the improvement? Probably all of these factors combine to bring about the favorable result. All that we know at present is that concomitant with the disappearance of the pain and hyperesthesia there is a loss of the coldness and sweating, and an improvement in muscle function of the affected part.

These observations are not unique. Leriche [64] has reported many cases of this type, and Kellgren [59] mentions some of them that were successfully treated by novocaine injection of an irritative focus. Dalton [13] states that he has cured pain syndromes of long standing by injection of novocaine solution into local areas of tenderness, and Homans [54] has reported a most interesting series of cases. These clinical observations must be accepted as factual even though an adequate physiologic explanation of the facts is not yet available.

## CHAPTER VII

## Post-traumatic Pain Syndromes

The cases classified as "post-traumatic pain syndromes" represent a symptom-complex characterized by severe pain and protracted disability following an apparently minor injury. Except that the pain lacks the "burning" quality that the term "causalgia" implies, they seem to be identical in type with the minor causalgias. They constitute the most numerous and most important representatives of that group of cases, ascribable to chronic irritation of sensory nerve fibers, which I have termed "the causalgic states." The fact that they are described separately gives me an opportunity to discuss some other aspects of the general problems created by the causalgic states, than have been mentioned in the previous two chapters.

Cases of this type have been reported in the medical literature for many generations, and it was appreciated long ago that they arose because of injuries to nerves. In the days when "bleeding" was an almost universal method for treating illness, the lancet wound to open a vein sometimes led to severe pain and muscular contractures that were known as "bent arm." Such an accident occurred to Charles IX, and the case was reported by Ambroise Paré [94] (p. 401) "for the edification of young surgeons." King Charles was stricken with a fever, and after a consultation, it was decided that he should be bled. A barber with a good reputation for successful bleedings was called in. As the vein was opened, a nerve was pricked. The King immediately cried out, complaining of great pain, and at the same time his arm contracted suddenly and strongly. Various remedies were applied but for more than three months the King was unable to flex or extend his arm. At the end of this time he recovered with only a moderate loss of strength in the arm. Paré evidently considered injuries of this kind to be serious in their consequences, for he comments that if the remedies he employed had not been sufficient to bring about a cure, he would not have hesitated to use boiling oil in the wound, or to have cut the nerve completely. He stated that it seemed to him more expedient to sacrifice the usefulness of the arm than to let the King perish miserably for want of doing it.

Fortunately, such instances of pain and disability after minor wounds are rare. They occur more commonly after war wounds than they do in civil life, but there are a sufficient number of them seen in industrial clinics to give them importance. It is likely that many of them will turn up during the present world conflict because of the large number of wounds due to shell fragments. It would be highly desirable if cases of this type could be grouped together in a base hospital. Careful study of such a group would not only mean better treatment and shorter disability periods for these wounded men, but should throw light on this whole subject.

In the industrial clinic the "post-traumatic pain syndromes" constitute a serious problem. They are difficult to recognize and difficult to cure. The subjective complaints appear to be excessive both as regards the spontaneous pain and the local hyperesthesia, because the causative injury may be innocuous in appearance and x-ray studies fail to show bone injury. The distribution of the pain frequently does not conform to definite peripheral nerve patterns. The coldness, cyanosis and edema may be ascribed to immobilization of the extremity in the dependent position. Tests for muscle strength elicit responses that seem inconsistent with the degree of atrophy and the apparent condition of the musculature. The examiner may conclude that pain prevents the patient from giving his full cooperation, or may decide that he is exaggerating or malingering. When with this clinical picture there is an accompanying "nervousness," excessive sweating, tremor and rapid pulse, it is not unnatural to ascribe the condition to a psychoneurosis or a "compensation neurosis."

A word concerning compensation is in order. Most of the workmen in this country are protected by some form of industrial insurance, which provides for their medical and hospital care, the payment of a percentage of their customary wages during the period of disability, and some form of monetary award for any permanent partial disability that may remain at the time the case is closed. The good features of this protection are, to some degree, offset by the fact that it provides a financial incentive for the workman who does not want to work because he is lazy or physically unfit, and for the workman who is inclined to malinger. Only a physician who has personally observed the difficulties encountered in the closure of claims during times when work is scarce and wages low, as compared to those in which wages are high and the demand for workmen exceeds the supply, as at present, can fully appreciate what these monetary incentives mean. The physician who has this personal experience cannot escape the gradual acquisition of an attitude of suspicion toward the workman whose complaints seem to be disproportionate to the apparent extent of his injury. He may come to feel that true malingering is not common, but he sees enough of it to give him a constant awareness of this possibility in every case he examines. He sees a much greater number of workmen who consciously or unconsciously exaggerate their suffering and the degree of disability, in the hope of being given a higher permanent disability award when their claim is closed. Therefore, when he encounters a case of post-traumatic pain syndrome, his first reaction is one of suspicion. The complaints seem to be out of all proportion to the original trauma. Yet accompanying the complaints there are objective evidences of a reflex dystrophy which his experience has taught him cannot be disregarded.

It sounds anomalous to say that an examination by a physician who has been made so aware of malingering and exaggeration offers the surest protection of the workman against a wrong evaluation of his case. Yet I believe this is true. Physicians with a long experience in industrial surgery are much less likely to underestimate the reality of irritative nerve lesions and reflex dystrophies, no matter how bizarre may be their manifestations, than are the best of the orthopedic specialists and neurosurgeons who may lack that particular background training. The examining physician may not be able to say just why he believes that the complaints are real; he may have no explanation as to how an apparently trivial injury can bring about such widespread reflex changes; but he has seen a sufficient number of cases that are so similar that he is unable to escape the conviction that there is an underlying physiologic disturbance in all of them.

To recognize an instance of post-traumatic pain syndrome is not as difficult as it is to cure the condition. The usual forms of physiotherapy either produce no lasting benefit, or may actually make the suffering worse. Many cases cannot tolerate any form of heat, and often the affected part is so hyperesthetic that massage and active exercise are prohibited. Sometimes a trigger point is found that is accessible for surgical excision, or its sensitiveness may be abolished by repeated injections of novocaine. Injections may be confined to the region of a suspected trigger point or may be aimed at blocking the impulses carried by the major nerves supplying the affected area, or in cases with obvious vasomotor phenomena, a considerable measure of relief may be afforded by injecting the appropriate sympathetic ganglia. Such injections may be successful in interrupting the reflexes responsible for, or contributing to, the pain syndrome. If they are successful, the hyperesthesia disappears and coincidentally the pains are alleviated, not only those ascribed to the trigger zone, but also pains felt at a considerable distance away in the distribution of other major nerves. Not infrequently there is also a remarkable increase in the muscle strength and the mobility of nearby joints. With these changes there is an associated improvement in the local circulation as evidenced by warming and changes in color of the part.

If such an attack on this causalgic state is instituted early, a single treatment may establish a cure. In long-established cases a similar dramatic cure occasionally occurs after one injection, but ordinarily the reflex disturbance is difficult to dispel, and several injections, at one or more of the points of attack that have been suggested, are required to bring about a lasting cure.

Case No. 9.—Mr. M. G., a 32-year-old truck driver struck the ulnar side of his right forearm against the end-gate of his truck. X-rays did not reveal a fracture and the local discoloration and swelling did not last long. But he complained of constant pain which was not relieved by physiotherapy treatments carried out for many months. He complained of weakness in the grip of the right hand and a tendency to drop things. He stated that when he drank a cup of coffee he had to hold the left hand under the cup for fear he would unexpectedly drop it. The whole arm was said to ache, and the hand was cold and often of a dusky color. He said the forearm and hand felt "half asleep and numb."

Examining physicians had told the insurance carriers that they found no objective evidence of anything wrong with the hand and arm except for a slight coldness. The officials of the insurance company were convinced that he "didn't want to return to work," but his family physician, who had known the man for years, was equally insistent that "something was still wrong." Examination showed that there was an accurately localized spot of tenderness remaining at the site of his original injury, and when a few cubic centimeters of 2 per cent novocaine solution had been infiltrated into this area there was an immediate improvement in the strength of his grip and a disappearance of his pain. The arm was "sore" for a few days after the injection but the pain did not return and within a week he was back at work.

CASE No. 10.—Mrs. G. E. B., a housewife, aged 54, fell against a door in her own home in November, 1938. The right upper arm was struck and a local ecchymosis developed, but the injury was not considered serious enough to require the services of a physician. It was not until two months later that she became aware of a sharp pain in the original area, that came on when she had her arm in certain positions. She consulted a physician, who took an x-ray plate. There was no evidence of bone injury. She received large doses of Vitamin B and diathermy treatments and finally spent a month in the hospital with hot packs on the arm and shoulder. But she seemed to get worse. Her pain was particularly severe at night. There was an increasing stiffness of the shoulder, and the arm felt "half asleep and cold all the time." She was unable to do her housework because any exercise aggravated her pain and hurt her stiff shoulder. The arm could not be laterally abducted more than forty degrees from her side; there was almost no rotation at the shoulder and she could not get her fingers to her face. The most tender part of the arm seemed to be a deep-lying transverse "band" just below the insertion of the deltoid, that was about two inches in length and a half inch wide. This band would suggest a tightly contracted group of muscle fibers were it not that no fibers normally run in this direction at that particular spot. Between June 6th and September 26th, 1939, she received eight injections of novocaine into this area. The injections were carried out at increasing intervals. The band gradually disappeared and within the first month she could touch the top of her head with her fingers. With the pain gone she could use an overhead pulley to stretch the tight shoulder muscles and by the middle of September had a normal range of motion at the shoulder. There was no recurrence of symptoms.

CASE No. 11.—Mr. D. A. B., a man of 32, complaining of severe pain in his left foot, was examined in January, 1932. Thirteen years previously this foot had become swollen and painful just proximal to the metatarsal heads. He had been exercising daily in a gymnasium but did not recall any specific injury to the foot. The pain gradually increased in severity, the foot was cold, atrophied and damp with sweat, while the ankle joint stiffened. The extensor tendons of all of the toes began to shorten until the toes were pulled upward onto the dorsum of the foot. When he walked, the ball of his foot felt as if he were "walking on a chunk of ice," and the toes would become blue and very cold. In 1920 a tendon-lengthening operation was done without mitigating the pain, and within a few months the toes were again displaced upward. He drifted from hospital to hospital seeking relief. He submitted to a double radical sinus operation, and his tonsils, appendix and all his teeth were removed. He obtained moderate relief from hot baths and liquor.

At the time of examination in 1932, the foot and leg were atrophied, the skin thin, shiny and damp with perspiration. The toes were drawn upward and the small joints of the foot were stiff and sensitive to manipulation. The entire foot was cold and hyperesthetic. The lateral aspect of the dorsum of the foot seemed to be the most hyperesthetic area, and touching this part brought on severe pain and a clonic jerking of the entire extremity, which he could not control.

An injection of novocaine in the region of the left lumbar sympathetic ganglia brought a prompt warming of the foot and relief from pain. On the basis of this test a lumbar ganglionectomy was carried out on the left side. The result was very satisfactory, and a year later he returned requesting that a similar operation be carried out on the right side. He had not complained of the right foot during his previous hospital stay, but he explained that the mild symptoms in the right foot which had been present for some years before 1932, had been overshadowed by those of the left foot. The symptoms ascribed to the right foot were identical in quality and localization with those originally felt on the left side, but except for a slight shortening of the extensor tendons of the toes, physical signs were not obvious. A right lumbar ganglionectomy was carried out. At the last follow-up examination in December, 1937, both feet were found to be warm, dry and comfortable. The atrophy of the tissues and drawing-up of the toes had disappeared and he walked normally. He had been working regularly. There had been a striking improvement in his weight, facial expression and emotional stability.

The point of immediate interest in this case is the reflection of the same signs and symptoms, though to a lesser degree, in the contralateral extremity. It is noted that after years of trouble in the left foot, he began to have an exactly similar trouble in the right foot. While this "reflected" symptom complex remained overshadowed by the more severe pain from the left side, he neglected to mention it, but even after the original syndrome had been abolished, the "mirror image" involving the right side persisted. The patient considered his symptoms serious enough to make him willing to undergo a second major operation to secure relief.

## MIRROR IMAGES

This remarkable tendency for a long-established pain syndrome to spread to involve the contralateral limb has been observed in some thirty-five cases I have personally examined. In rare instances it is the ipsolateral limb that reflects the original trouble, but in such instances the mirroring is less obvious. The term "mirror image" is justified by the striking similarity shown by the process as it spreads to the contralateral limb. If the original injury involves the right great toe, it is the left great toe that is primarily involved in the reflecting disturbance. If vasomotor phenomena are prominent in the original syndrome, there are vasomotor changes of lesser degree on the opposite side. Pain and hyperesthesia are more likely to characterize the "mirror" phenomena, than are the more objective signs of vasomotor disturbance, muscle changes and edema, but all of these have been observed. The signs and symptoms are never as prominent as in the area of original involvement, even in those cases that are considered as typical "mirror images." And in a surprisingly large number of additional cases, the patient is sufficiently aware of the reflection of pain to the normal limb to cause him to fear that his trouble is "going over to the other side."

Weir Mitchell [85] made frequent note of mirror images, although he did not employ this term. As examples (p. 305), in discussing a case with causalgia in the right hand, he says: "The left hand, which, it will be remembered, was also eczematous, is painful on pressure and touch, especially in the palm. He is positive that there is pain in that hand, and that it is a burning pain." Again, in discussing skin changes in the causalgic states he writes (p. 159): "Since our report, Mr. Annandale has published a very interesting history of wound of a finger, with tender cicatrix, followed by glossy redness of the skin of the same hand, and finally of the opposite hand. Mr. Syme removed the finger, which soon relieved the hand first involved, but was succeeded by swelling and increase of pain in the other hand. The history, unfortunately, ends here, and there was no microscopic examination of the portion of the nerves removed. This is especially to be regretted, because of the mystery which hangs over the production of this form of mal-nutrition of skin and its accompanying pain. I have never seen any distinct redness or swelling upon the opposite side, although in several examples the sense of burning and the hyperesthetic state of the skin was apt to affect first the symmetrically related member, and then other regions of the whole surface. In a single instance, the unwounded limb was attacked by a vesicular eruption like that which existed on the other side."

Sometimes there is a mirrored complaint of muscle "cramps" or a constant muscle "tightness" and in some instances a noticeable shortening of the tendons becomes apparent. Although the involvement of muscles and tendons is much less common than pain and hyperesthesia, in rare cases the motor phenomena of the mirror image constitute a more striking feature than are the sensory changes. This rare type of mirror image is illustrated by the following case.

CASE No. 12.—Mr. W. B. was seen in consultation at the Veterans' Hospital in 1938 to decide on the advisability of amputation of the leg, or some other procedure to relieve him of persistent burning pain in the left foot. In 1926 he fell off a submarine and his left leg was struck by the propeller. He sustained a compound, comminuted fracture of both bones of the lower leg about four inches above the ankle joint. Infection developed. The leg was saved but was of questionable value to him because of marked deformity and a persistent burning pain in the middle three toes. The great toe and little toe were largely spared, but the second, third and fourth toes felt as if they were on fire, and gradually began to pull back over the dorsum of the foot. The patient stated that by the end of a year after the accident these three toes were "upside down" on top of the foot, while his first and fifth toes remained in their usual position. In 1930 he noticed that the same three toes of the right foot were beginning to draw up. He does not recall that there was much, or any, pain in the right foot, but admits that he may have been too much diverted by the burning pain in the left foot to notice. In the course of a few months the middle three toes were "almost as deformed as the same three toes of the left foot" and he could no longer wear a shoe on this foot unless the top was cut away. The great toe and little toe of the right foot remained in their usual position. In 1933 a surgeon removed the three middle toes of the left foot in the hope of getting rid of the burning pain. At the same time he removed the same three toes of the right foot so that the man could wear an ordinary shoe, explaining to the patient at that time that the right toes had drawn up "in sympathy" with the left toes. At the time of our examination, then, all six toes were gone, so we had no opportunity to make comparisons. The great toes and little toes of the two sides were normal in posture. There was no complaint of pain or hyperesthesia relating to the right foot, but the left foot was still the seat of a terrible burning, chiefly ascribed to the three "phantom" toes. This pain was relieved following amputation above the level of the old injury.

The tendency for signs and symptoms to spread to the opposite limb is a significant observation. It is not confined to the post-traumatic pain syndrome cases, but seems to be a characteristic of all of the "causalgic states." It might be said that the tendency to "spread" is the most important feature of these states. The reflex disturbance first spreads beyond the distributions of the sensory nerve originally involved by the irritative lesion; then it may spread to the opposite limb, to an ipsilateral limb, or even to affect the functioning of one whole side of the body.

Of even greater significance, perhaps, is the observation that once a new area is involved in a disturbance of function, the process may continue after the original lesion has lost its sustaining effect. It is difficult to escape the conviction that some dynamic process has been initiated within the spinal cord that may persist after the original stimulus is withdrawn. Such a possibility is intriguing because it suggests that the original irritative lesion initiates some change in the activities of the regulatory centers of the central nervous system that eventually acquires a self-sustaining momentum.

I do not expect that such an interpretation will be accepted by the reader at its face value. There will be subsequent opportunities to refer to it again, and to offer experimental evidence that seems to favor this concept of a dynamic central agency separate from, and eventually independent of, the original irritant focus. I mention it now so that the reader will have it in mind as he reads the remainder of this monograph, and to indicate my belief that it is through the activities of this central agency that the bizarre extensions of the causalgic states may take place. We are accustomed to thinking of any spread of activity within the spinal cord in terms of anatomic proximity. For instance, we know that visceral disease often expresses itself in distant areas. Ureteral colic may give rise to pain ascribed to the penis, the testicle and the inner side of the thigh; the testicle may become sensitive to any contact, and often is retracted by a contraction of the dartos muscle; and the skin of the thigh near the groin may become hyperesthetic. These are "referred phenomena," occurring in tissues far from the irritant lesion, that we have come to accept as commonplace, just as we accept the reference of pain and hyperesthesia down a particular part of the left arm in angina pectoris; or the spread of pain in angina to the right arm, and the sensation of pain ascribed to the normal kidney when the actual lesion is on the opposite side. But despite the fact that the referred phenomena appear in areas distant from the lesion, it is usually possible to demonstrate that the irritant impulses from the dis- eased viscus involve the same segments of the spinal cord as do the impulses concerned in the referred phenomena.

Because such interpretations have become commonplace in clinical interpretations, we do not hesitate to accept the reality of referred pain so long as it can be shown that there exists a segmental relationship between the causative lesion and the area of reference. But when the pain is referred to some spot that has no segmental relationship with the irritant focus our tendency is to immediately question its reality. Let me men- tion a few common examples. For instance, a man who has had an injury to his lower back, complains that the pain ascends upward along one side of his spine, up over his head to involve the eye region of the affected side. The medical examiner sees no segmental relationship between the areas involved in such a spread of symptoms, and therefore is inclined to question its reality. But when this same reference of symptoms is reported again and again by other patients he may not be so dogmatic in his denial of its reality. Or if he submits to an injection of a small amount of hypertonic salt solution into the erector muscles of his own back, as Kellgren and Lewis [70] have done, he will observe that the spread of pain and muscle spasm actu- ally does extend up and down the back far beyond the limits of any single spinal segment. Many individuals have discov- ered that the stimulation of certain parts of their body may give rise to sensations in distant parts which have no obvious anatomic relationship to the area stimulated. I can invariably elicit a tingling sensation directly over the medial condyle of my left humerus by scratching a small area at the anterior costal margin. A friend tells me that the stimulation of a particular spot on his knee will cause a sharp, stinging pain on his anterior chest wall. Just why or how such "facilitated" pathways between two segmentally unrelated parts of the body come to be established is not known, but that such connections exist cannot be questioned.

## CHAPTER VIII

## *Chronic Low Back Disability*

In the last chapter attention was called to the fact that an irritable focus at the periphery may initiate a dynamic process involving the regulatory centers of the nervous system. It was suggested that through the agency of this central process reflexes tended to spread to neighboring and even distant parts of the body. A quite similar mechanism is called into play in certain cases of chronic back disability, and I should like to briefly consider some of the aspects of such cases as they relate to the principal theme of the monograph. It should be clearly understood that I am not undertaking a discussion of the whole complex subject of low back disability, nor am I advocating a particular method of treatment for the many different kinds of back pain.

Sometimes a simple lifting strain may start the pathologic process that results in protracted disability. A workman that has long been accustomed to lifting heavy boxes, happens to lift a relatively light one while making a turn, and experiences during this exertion a "catch" in his lower back. For a moment the pain is sharp and the workman may drop the box. When the acute pain has passed, a dull ache, accurately localized at the site of the original pain, may persist, but frequently this is not sufficient to prevent his continuing his work for hours or even days after the accident. The workman is not particularly concerned over the ache and may not report an accident, expecting that the slight discomfort will disappear spontaneously as other minor discomforts have done in the past. Instead, the ache persists and the pain which has only been mildly annoying and accurately localized, becomes more intense and widespread. It may now seem to come from the back, the buttock and the back of the thigh and leg, even down into the foot. Nerve trunks may become sensitive to pressure. Muscle spasm develops that is no longer confined to the region of the original injury, and the spastic muscles not only fail to respond readily to command, but become new sources for pain. The extremity into which the pain is referred may be cold, damp with perspiration, and the site of local areas of paresthesia. The workman may complain that in addition to the ache extending into the leg there is a feeling of numbness, formication or a sensation "as if water were running down the leg."

As this process spreads it becomes increasingly difficult to identify the location and the nature of the original lesion. What started as a simple low back sprain now becomes classified as a "sciatica," or a "myofascitis" ascribed to parts at a considerable distance from the original trouble. At this stage there is usually no question of the workman continuing on the job. He is compelled to lay off work because of a very real disability. It is most difficult to predict how long the period of disability will be in such a case, and I have seen men laid off work for months and years as a result of what seemed to have been a very trivial accident. In fact, the observation that impressed me most in the several years I served as a Medical Examiner for the Oregon State Industrial Accident Commission, was that there was no reliable parallelism between the period of disability and the apparent severity of the original accident, in the cases of low back disability taken as a whole. This is not to say that serious accidents attended by bone and joint injury may not have warranted a more serious prognosis than the simple lifting strains. It simply records the fact that in certain instances the period of disability following what seemed to have been a minor accident sometimes far exceeded that resulting from much more severe injuries.

One of the remarkable features of many cases of low back disability, is the tendency for the attacks to recur after long intervals of relative freedom from signs and symptoms. Once in a while a case is encountered that proves to be resistant to the usual methods of treatment, but suddenly gets well after a fall or some sudden movement. A still larger number may date the beginning of their recovery from symptoms to some manipulation of their backs.

I have had a personal experience with low back pain which undoubtedly influences my reaction to "manipulations." I have suffered four or five attacks of pain which seemed to originate in my left sacroiliac joint region. Each attack has been brought on during physical exercise such as bowling or playing badminton. It starts with a sudden, sharp pain, sometimes accompanied by a "snap." The sharp pain is transient, but afterward there is a persistent dull discomfort ascribed to one very definite spot just below the posterior spine of the ilium. The discomfort at first is not sufficient to prevent my continuing the game, but the following morning my back is stiff and sore and I walk with a slight list. If left untreated, the trouble tends to increase, and at the end of a few days it is difficult to get out of a chair, or get in or out of my car. When I get up from a sitting posture it is impossible to at once come erect, and when walking there is an obvious stiffness and list to the back. I have to be assisted in dressing and am unable to put on my socks and shoes. My inability to bend down to my shoes is not determined alone by the pain the bending entails, because I have tried throwing my body weight forward with great force and have failed to reach that far. The muscle spasm, at first local, now involves the whole lower back, buttock and thigh, and in addition to the pain there is a feeling as if this whole area had been poured full of molten lead which hardened there. At this stage it is difficult to localize the pain accurately, the region being generally painful. Novocaine injections near the site from which the pain seems to originate afford temporary relief only. An unsuccessful manipulation of the back seems to aggravate the pain, but a successful one causes a snap that may be audible. When this occurs there is an immediate sense of relief, even though much of the pain and muscle spasm are still present. The residual muscle stiffness and soreness gradually disappear once the underlying source of irritation has been corrected, and within three or four days I am back playing badminton without the slightest back disability.

The story of the onset of the back pain, and the relief afforded by manipulation, combine to indicate that some anatomic change has occurred, or, as the layman puts it, "something slipped out of place," and the manipulation permitted it to "go back into place." To many physicians such a story would be interpreted as implicating an intervertebral disc, since this is the only structure capable of displacement and replacement, which has been actually demonstrated as an anatomic cause of back disability. It is perfectly possible that my case and many others that have been ascribed to "sacro-iliac slips" and other equally vague mechanisms, are in reality due to the displacement of an intervertebral disc. On the other hand, the exact localization of the original pain, and its correspondence to the area from which the snap seems to come, do not always support this assumption. However, the question toward which this discussion is leading, is not which of several different kinds of mechanical displacement might account for the syndrome, but how any of them may act to initiate the disturbance.

In the case of a displaced intervertebral disc the problem does not appear difficult. The most frequent location of the offending disc is at the fourth or fifth lumbar interspace. The disc slips forward to protrude into the spinal canal and in so doing presses on the nerve bundles of the cauda equina. It may come into direct contact with nerves of the sacral plexus so as to cause symptoms referred to the extremities. If the pressure is severe the nerve fibers cease to conduct impulses and there results a loss of reflexes, muscle atrophy and areas of diminished sensibility. If the pressure is insufficient to abolish nerve conduction, the contact may act to irritate the nerve fibers and thus give rise to disturbances of function of the muscles and paresthesias. The mechanics involved in the displacement and subsequent nerve pressure is obvious and a removal of the offending disc may lead to a prompt relief of symptoms.

Yet I am not sure that the emphasis placed on the mechanical aspects of this process is entirely justified. Certainly, a very similar series of functional disturbances can result from lesions in which mechanical pressures are not demonstrable. Kellgren's [59] observations bear on this point. He employs a 6 per cent solution of sodium chloride to inject into the muscles of volunteer subjects assisting in his investigations. The hypertonic solution causes an aching pain for a few seconds, but apparently does no permanent damage. Kellgren has shown that a few drops of this solution injected into the erector spinae muscle causes pain that does not remain confined to the site of injection but spreads up and down along the spine for several segments. He finds that a very few minims injected into one intercostal space may give rise to pain which is referred along that single interspace, while a greater quantity of the solution in the same area will cause a pain which spreads over several interspaces. The anatomy of the intercostal space would make it apparent that the spread of the pain could not be ascribed to a diffusion of the irritant fluid to the adjoining interspaces. Instead the spread must be dependent upon a neural reference.

Lewis and Kellgren [70] have used this same hypertonic saline in the study of pain reference from irritated intervertebral fascia. They report that a small amount injected into the intervertebral fascia at the first lumbar level gives rise to an aching pain that may simulate the pain of ureteral colic in its distribution. The pain is said to be accompanied by muscle spasm, both deep and superficial tenderness, and may even result in a spontaneous retraction of the testicle on the affected side. Here again, it is evident that the spread of signs and symptoms must depend upon reflexes set up by sensory nerve irritation, rather than upon any mechanical effects of the injection.

Steindler and Luck [112] have demonstrated that in a series of 451 patients suffering from low back pain, more than 20 per cent suffered from symptoms which they believed were reflex in origin, and not properly ascribable to a nerve root compression. In each of these cases it was possible to demonstrate a local point of tenderness situated in the distribution of the posterior division of the spinal nerves. The authors ascribed symptoms, referred to distant parts supplied by the anterior divisions of the spinal nerves, to these focal areas of tenderness, and were of the opinion that the lesions represented either a deep ligamentous injury or a myofascitis. They used novocaine injections of the local lesion to establish a causal relation between the trigger point and the radiating symptomatology. Five postulates had to be met before the relationship was considered proven:

1. Contact with the needle must aggravate the local pain.
2. Contact with the needle must elicit or aggravate radiation.
3. Procaine hydrochloride infiltration must suppress local tenderness.
4. Procaine hydrochloride infiltration must suppress radiation.
5. Positive leg signs must disappear.

Steindler and Luck were of the opinion that the actual percentage of cases of low back pain in which such a reflex disturbance from a single trigger point may take place, may be higher than they have reported, since "it is likely that some cases were missed because the involved area was not closely enough identified by the inserted needle." Even the 20 per cent is a remarkably high percentage to be found as meeting the exacting postulates they established. Of the 142 cases with the posterior division syndrome, 103 were treated satisfactorily by conservative methods, and 30 were subjected to surgical treatment because of the persistence of irritation from some lesion that was not eliminated by simple immobilization.

I have reported [75] a small series of cases that seem to represent the posterior division syndrome as described by Steindler and Luck, in which the trigger point was found to lie within a triangular zone on each side of the upper part of the sacrum. I have called this area the "multifidus triangle" because in it lies the lowermost portions of the multifidus muscle which acts to stabilize the spine in its relation to the sacrum. The extent of the triangle is shown in the accompanying figures. (Figs. 14, 15 and 16.)

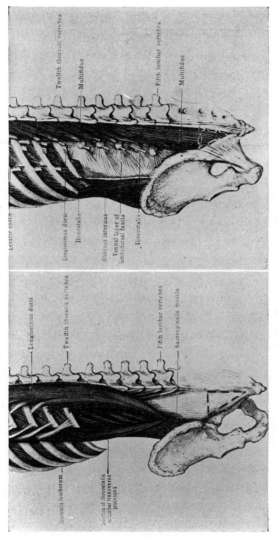

Fig. 14 — Longissimus dorsi
Twelfth thoracic vertebra
Fifth lumbar vertebra
Sacrospinalis muscle
Iliocostalis lumborum
Insertion of iliocostalis on lumbar transverse processes

Levator costæ
Twelfth thoracic vertebra
Multifidus
Longissimus dorsi
Iliocostalis
Obliquus internus
Ventral layer of lumbo-dorsal fascia
Iliocostalis
Fifth lumbar vertebra
Multifidus

FIGS. 14 AND 15.—THE MULTIFIDUS TRIANGLE

The dotted lines in these three figures indicate the general extent of the area which has been termed the "multifidus triangle." It represents an inverted right-angle triangle whose base extends from the midline to the posterior superior spine of the ileum, and whose apex is at the lowermost point of origin for the multifidus muscle.

Fig. 14 shows the fascia of the sacrospinal muscle, which forms a dense aponeurotic covering for the deeper structures within the triangle.

Fig. 15 shows the multifidus muscle after the sacrospinalis muscle and its fascia have been removed.

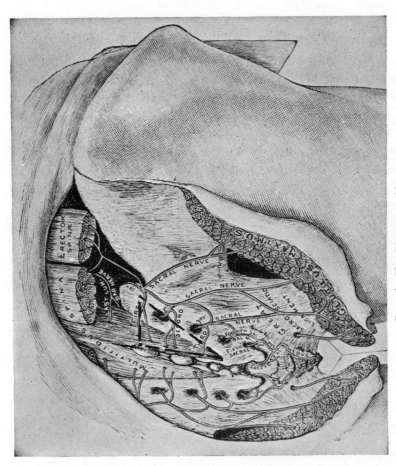

FIG. 16.—THE MULTIFIDUS TRIANGLE

Fig. 16 shows the posterior branches of the first, second and third sacral nerves that supply the structures within the multifidus triangle.

There are three different structures in this region which might be affected by an injection of novocaine solution. I am not including the skin and subcutaneous tissues as one of these because when the infiltration is limited to the superficial tissues a favorable response to injection is not obtained. The first structure that may be of importance is the aponeurosis of the sacrospinalis muscle, which has its origin from the lower part of the sacrum and spreads in a thick fascial sheet over the triangle. Beneath this fascia lies the multifidus muscle, its lowermost fibers representing the apex of the triangle, and forming a surprisingly wide and deep muscle mass toward the base of the triangle. I have had the impression that novocaine injections produced their best effects when they were made beneath the sacrospinalis fascia into the substance of the multifidus muscle. I have also been influenced to believe that the trigger point I am seeking may be represented by some injury to this muscle, because the original injury is usually produced during muscular effort when the body was bent forward at the hips.

The third structure which may be involved by the injection, and which unquestionably plays an important part in the pain syndrome, is nerve. Sensory fibers of the posterior division of the first, second and third sacral nerves are supplied to this triangular zone. Presumably, it is the filaments of these nerves which are irritated by the local lesion sufficiently to set up the secondary reflex disturbance.

In the cases suffering from the so-called "multifidus syndrome" of low back pain and disability, there is not only a demonstrable point of local tenderness, but pressure over the most sensitive point usually aggravates the pain and causes a typical reference of pain radiating out over the anterior divisions in the manner described in the history previously elicited.

If the patient has complained of pain extending into the lower leg along the course of the sciatic nerve, pressure over the tender spot may cause a sudden, sharp pain to shoot downward over this same course. If the pain has been ascribed to the lateral aspect of the thigh, then pressure may reproduce that reference. Some connection undoubtedly exists in each case, between the tender area and the region to which symptoms are referred, and this connection most probably is dependent upon central relationships because distant nerves may be involved as well as the anterior divisions of the nerve roots originally stimulated. The connection suggests that some particular pathway within the central nervous system had become "facilitated." The longer the pain continues, the more definitely established does the connection become. When the sensitiveness of the trigger point has been eliminated, the association is lost. The pain disappears, and with it go the motor reflexes responsible for the changes taking place in the muscles, sweat glands and blood vessels.

CASE No. 13.—Mr. L. W. B., aged 47, a brakeman on a donkey engine, was injured on April 16, 1938, when he was "jack-knifed" by a sudden lurch of the engine. He experienced a sudden pain to the left of the midline over the sacrum. The pain was so severe that he fainted. While in the hospital the pain spread out over the gluteal region and down the back of his left thigh to the popliteal space. The pain was described as being of a burning character, worse during stormy weather, and aggravated by any sudden movement, straining, sneezing, etc. He spent months in the hospital but the treatment did not materially diminish his pain. When I saw him in May, 1940, he was ambulatory, wearing a Taylor back brace with crutch supports, and which seemed to give his back some comfort. He was given eight injections of 2 per cent novocaine solution into a very sensitive spot in the left multifidus triangle. He was discharged as cured late in June and has been at work since.

CASE No. 14.—Miss M. H., aged 27, a librarian, slipped on wet pavement on April 9, 1938, and fell, striking on her lower back. She experienced a "sickening pain" and the sacral area felt "numb" for several days. Her work was not heavy, and in spite of persistent pain she continued at her job. She carried an air cushion to sit on, and when off work, as well as during her two weeks' vacation that summer, she spent her time in bed with heat on her back. During each menstrual period her pain was greatly aggravated, and it is of interest to note that she had always had painful periods, and that the pain was usually referred to this same portion of her lower back.

When I examined her first on November 22, 1938, she told me that all of the usual methods of treatment had been tried without alleviating her pain. There was a single exception to this statement. She had been given seven or eight injections of novocaine into the tissues over the sacrum, and although she felt that these injections tended to make her worse for three or more days after each treatment, one injection had given her complete relief for ten days. It was this story that made me think I could find a definite trigger point in her back. There were many tender areas over the sacrum and the coccyx, but the principal one was at the apex of the left multifidus triangle close to the midline. When this point had been injected three times all the other tender spots disappeared, her pain and disability were relieved and have not recurred.

It may be misleading to mention the "multifidus syndrome" in this discussion, because the impression might be left that this particular area is the only one in which trigger points are to be found. This is not true, trigger points being found frequently in the gluteus muscles, the pyriformis, or in any of the muscles or the fascia of the lower back and buttocks. Nor is it true that repeated novocaine injections will always be successful in establishing a cure of symptoms, no matter how favorable may be the immediate response to treatment. In many cases, particularly those in which some abnormal tension or mechanical pinching of tissues persists, it is not to be expected that treatment will do more than confer temporary relief. It is quite possible that treatment may succeed in breaking up the pathologic process for a time, but the factors which contributed to the onset of the trouble remain to start it all over again. Novocaine injections of sensitive points in the lower back are well worth trying both as a means for determining the source of pathologic reflexes, and as a method of treatment, but it is not a panacea, merely a useful adjunct to other methods of treatment.

My principal interest in the method is quite aside from its therapeutic usefulness. It serves to demonstrate the central thesis of this monograph, i.e., that a peripherally situated trigger point is capable of initiating a pathologic state characterized by spreading reflexes, and probably dependent upon a disturbed physiologic status of the spinal centers. I would emphasize the physiologic nature of certain instances of the syndrome of low back disability. I am inclined to believe that even in the cases which do not respond favorably to injection therapy, and which may represent more extensive organic involvement, the irritation of sensory nerve filaments and the secondary reflex mechanism which results from the persistent irritation, plays an important role in the development of the low back syndrome. In other words, while I do not disregard the importance of the anatomical and mechanical aspects of bone and joint injury in the production of the disability, I believe that the principal factor in determining the degree of disability a particular lesion may entail is not measured solely by the visible evidences of injury, but by the manner in which such a lesion happens to irritate sensory nerve filaments. Perhaps the situation is not dissimilar to that observed when nerve trunks are cut, crushed, or compressed. In many instances such injuries to nerves do not set up a causalgic state, and are attended by no unusual degree of pain or disability. Yet under conditions that are not clear, an exactly similar nerve lesion may cause severe pain and start the spreading reflex disturbance recognized as causalgia.

## CHAPTER IX

## Facial Neuralgias

It is with considerable hesitation that I venture to mention trigger mechanisms as they may relate to pain in the head and face. To a large extent this hesitancy springs from my own uncertainties. I am confused by the terms that are used to designate the varied kinds of headache and neuralgic pains occurring in the face and neck. I am baffled by the post-traumatic headaches, "migraine," and the "vascular neuralgias." I am frequently at a loss to know how to treat some of my cases, and my efforts fail too frequently to qualify me to speak with assurance on this subject. Many of the patients I am called upon to treat are derelicts in the sense that they have been abandoned by their physicians after the usual methods of treatment have failed. Often their teeth have been extracted, their sinuses and middle ears treated, their tonsils removed, and sometimes one or more of the nerves of the face or scalp have been divided without any permanent benefit.

The syndrome of major trigeminal neuralgia, though it probably represents the most severe and trying type of facial pain, constitutes much less of a problem than the minor or "atypical" neuralgias. The classical syndrome is not difficult to recognize, and its treatment is well standardized and effectual. Alcohol injection of the divisions of the fifth nerve, when skillfully done, usually confers relief for months or years. More certain and permanent is the relief afforded by a section of the fifth nerve root or an intramedullary tractotomy.[109] The effectiveness of treatment that is available for patients suffering from major trigeminal neuralgia serves to remove them from the problem group of "atypical neuralgias" which are the surgeon's chief concern. Yet it is true that little more is known of the actual etiology of major trigeminal neuralgia than of the minor forms. I must confess to an uncertainty as to how to classify some of my cases whose symptoms resemble those characterizing the classical syndrome, nor am I sure that the distinction which is customarily made between the major and minor types is significant of any fundamental difference in the mechanisms that underlie them. I have observed the disappearance of symptoms which could well be classified as trigeminal tic after the correction of a malocclusion, the effective treatment of a local area of "myositis" in the masseter muscle, and after repeated novocaine injections of trigger points.

It does not follow from these isolated observations, however, that major trigeminal neuralgia is ascribable to peripheral lesions nor that it will yield to conservative measures. The best evidence to the contrary is afforded by the great number of patients who have submitted to the removal of teeth and the treatment of foci of possible infection without relief from their pain. All that such observations can mean at present is that certain instances of "symptomatic neuralgia" may resemble major trigeminal neuralgia in the character of the pain paroxysms.

My sole purpose in mentioning facial neuralgias in this monograph is to call attention to the fact that trigger points may develop in the face, neck or scalp just as they do in the extremities or in the back; that they seem to be as capable of initiating pathologic reflexes as are other trigger points; and the fact that they sometimes yield to simple measures suggests that irritation from peripheral sources may play some part in the development of pain syndromes involving the head areas. I should like to avoid the controversial subject of classification, and the obscurities of the problem of etiology for facial pain in its various forms.

One of the most interesting types of trigger point that may give rise to pain is represented by small, palpable masses that are designated by the term "myositis." It is well known that a form of headache may develop secondary to the appearance of discrete kernels at the base of the skull and in the upper part of the neck. Sometimes the nodules seem to be deep in the muscle, sometimes they feel as if they were in the subcutaneous tissues. They are tender to pressure, so that massage may be painful, but this form of treatment may be most effective in dispelling their tenderness. Under massage, baking and counter-irritation they usually disappear, and with them goes the headache. Headaches of this type are classed as "indurative" headache, yet it is hardly justifiable to say that there is one kind of pain that characterizes them. The pain may be represented by an occipital ache, a generalized throbbing headache, or it may simulate the unilateral pain of migraine. Patients who have long suffered from indurative headache learn to recognize as signs of an impending attack, an increased sensitiveness of the nodules, and a feeling of stiffness of the neck muscles. Occasionally they can prevent an incapacitating headache from developing by local treatment that dispels the tenderness of the palpable masses.

Similar local areas of "myositis" developing in the temporal or masseter muscles may be responsible for facial pains. The tiny nodules may be difficult to find, particularly when they occur in the anterior margin of the masseter muscle. The muscle elsewhere may be stimulated without eliciting a pain response, but when this discrete kernel is pressed upon, a lancinating pain is felt in the lip, in the temporal region, or over the distribution of one or more divisions of the fifth nerve. Usually the pain they engender tends to be dull and persistent, but in severe cases the pain may occur in paroxysms that are identical with those of major trigeminal neuralgia, even to the facial grimace. Treatment by baking and massage will usually cause the nodules to disappear, and, simultaneously, the pain attacks cease. It is of interest to note that the first few treatments may aggravate the pain, while persistence in the same treatment is usually rewarded by a cure of the pain within two to six weeks.

More commonly the trigger point is not represented by a palpable mass. A point of deep tenderness in the scalp, in the gums or in the superficial layers of the skin may be found as the trigger point, without there being any other indication of a local pathology. Those that are found in the scalp are prone to occur over the course of the major and minor occipital nerves. Tapping lightly over such a local area of tenderness may elicit a pain radiating out over the peripheral distribution of the nerve. The pain may be described as a tingling soreness, a deep ache or as lancinating pain that comes in paroxysms like an electric shock. Not infrequently the scalp is sensitive to light contact for wide areas around the actual trigger point, the hairs may feel as if they were rumpled and stiffly protruding from the scalp. Shocks of pain may occur without an appreciable stimulus, causing the subject to wince and grimace each time they come. Similar trigger points may occur anywhere on the face, the commonest location being just lateral to the nasal ala. The pain may involve the distribution of one or more divisions of the fifth nerve, its tendency being to spread from the region of the trigger zone with the progress of the syndrome. When the condition has been present for a long time, the whole side of the face may seem to be hypersensitive, and the shocks may be precipitated by the slightest movement of the face muscles, a draft of wind, emotional states or minor variations in the environmental temperature.

CASE No. 15.—Mr. R. S., aged 58, suffered from occipital headaches for eight years. The pain always started on the left side of the head, behind the ear, and there was an associated tenderness of the scalp. Five years before I saw him, the major occipital nerve on the left side had been sectioned. The operation conferred partial relief for a period of weeks. The pain gradually increased to its original intensity while the area of distribution of the occipital nerve was still "completely numb." The return of sensation was never complete. The hair in this area felt "as if it were sticking straight out," and at times the scalp was exquisitely tender. Even when the pains were least severe, contact of the hairs with a pillow was "most disagreeable, though not exactly painful," and certain spots could be found, which, when pressed upon, caused a shock-like pain to dart up over the top of the head. Spontaneous paroxysms of these "shock-like" pains usually preceded a bad headache. The headache seemed to start in the left side of the neck and base of the skull and spread from there over the head. They were increased by fatigue and nervous tension. A series of novocaine injections during a three weeks' period reduced the local sensitiveness and abolished the headache for a month. Subsequent injections of the scar and two other trigger points conferred periods of complete relief that lasted for a month or six weeks at a time. This patient still requires additional injections at variable intervals to control his headaches.

CASE No. 16.—Miss B. L., aged 38, was referred for the investigation of headaches associated with a periodic itching and burning sensation in the left side of her scalp. She had been in an automobile accident eighteen months previously in which she sustained a fractured femur, a fractured jaw and a laceration above her left eye. For about six months after the accident the left side of her forehead and scalp had been numb. When sensation returned, the skin was hyperesthetic and she experienced attacks of intolerable itching. If she scratched the scalp, a severe burning sensation supervened which might last for hours, sometimes persisting all night. Coincident with the onset of the hyperesthesia she began to suffer from recurrent headache. The ache seemed to start in the left frontal region and spread to the temples, then to involve the whole head. In the year, they had increased in severity and frequency. In addition, she complained that she could not lie on her left side because it brought on dizziness and a sensation as if she were whirling in space in a clockwise direction. The scalp in the left frontal region was hyperesthetic but lacked the elevation of the tactile threshold and the impaired discrimination that often accompany the hyperesthetic state. Tapping or pressing over the scar at the supra-orbital notch gave rise to more complaint than when done over the peripheral portions of the supra-orbital nerve distribution.

Between December 9 and January 3, 1937, she was given four injections of novocaine into the scar just above the supra-orbital notch. After each injection there was a temporary increase in the local sensitiveness, followed by increasingly long periods of relief from headache, itching and burning. On February 23 she reported that she had had some itching of the scalp and a slight temporal headache, but this was the last recurrence of her symptoms.

An interesting sidelight on this young woman's history was the fact that her fiancé was killed in the same accident that produced her original injuries. The emotional crisis occasioned by his death, combined with the suffering and expense to which she was subjected during a long period of hospitalization, would have threatened the equilibrium of any normal person. When she returned to work and the headaches became so severe that she was losing more and more time from her job, it was not unnatural for her associates and her physician to assume that her complaints had a psychic origin. But there were many features of the case which made her physician hesitate to make this assumption. Her history suggested that the supra-orbital nerve had been cut; her complaints did not develop until there was evidence that the nerve was growing back through the scar; and her symptoms of itching, burning and headache, all seemed to originate in the involved area. And as he observed her efforts to continue her work in spite of increasing headache, he rejected the assumption. He came to the conclusion that her complaints had their origin in the scar above her left eye, a conclusion that was borne out by the response to treatment.

CASE No. 17.—Mrs. J. W., aged 78, had suffered for more than ten years with a trigeminal neuralgia involving the right side of her face. She recalled that the first sign of trouble was a sensitive spot above her right eye. When this was touched, a twinge of pain shot out over the distribution of the ophthalmic division of the fifth nerve. Later the maxillary division was involved and at times the pain was also felt in the lower jaw. The effect of the lancinating pain was sometimes so severe that she was unable to eat or talk. Examination showed that she had two trigger zones. The most sensitive one was located about three-quarters of an inch to the right of the midline and an equal distance above the margin of the orbit. It was very accurately localized and even light cotton-wool stimulation precipitated pain attacks. She seemed to tolerate light touch in this area less well than firm pressure. She had a second trigger zone in the region of the nasal ala, but this spot did not seem to be so accurately localized or so sensitive, although lancinating attacks of pain could be elicited by stimulation of this region. On September 13, 1938, I infiltrated the trigger zone of her forehead with 2 per cent novocaine. Following the injection I was unable to elicit pain by local pressure, but the supra-orbital nerve just below this point seemed to be slightly sensitive to pressure. I therefore supplemented the injection by an infiltration of the nerve at the supra-orbital notch. Peculiarly enough, these injections seemed to diminish the sensitiveness of the trigger zone near the nose, at least I could not thereafter precipitate an attack of pain by stimulating it. Four days later she reported that she had had a few mild attacks of pain in the ophthalmic distribution but none in the maxillary or mandibular divisions. Again I could not elicit pain by stimulation of the region of the nasal ala, but stimulation of the upper trigger zone on the forehead caused paroxysmal pain. This area was again infiltrated with a few minims of 2 per cent novocaine. This second injection was followed by nine days of complete relief and she said: "I feel like this is a different existence than I've had for the past ten years." I could elicit slight complaint of tenderness by direct pressure over the supra-orbital notch but could not precipitate an attack. She was given four injections, the last one on October 18, 1938, after which she had no pain for six months. In April, 1939, she experienced a few twinges of pain in the maxillary division, which seemed to originate just lateral to the nose and spread in shock-like reverberations over the cheek and upper jaw. There was no complaint of pain in the supra-orbital region at that time. One injection was given at the secondary trigger zone near the nose, and at the time of her last examination, eleven months after the final injection, there has been no recurrence of pain.

CASE No. 18.—Mr. J. M., aged 64, suffered from attacks of trigeminal neuralgia in 1932. In 1933 a competent neurosurgeon partially divided the posterior root of the fifth nerve using a subtemporal approach. He was completely relieved of pain for three years. Then, in spite of the fact that there was numbness in the distribution of the mandibular and maxillary divisions, the attacks, exactly similar in type, recurred. A second operation was carried out to divide the posterior root more completely. Again he had a period of three years of complete relief. In 1939 the pain attacks again began, in all respects similar to his previous trouble. He was advised to submit to a third operation, this time by a posterior approach to divide the posterior root closer to its brain connection. He refused the third operation. At the time of my first examination in May, 1940, he said that his pain was beyond description, in spite of large doses of

hypnotics and opiates. Eating, smoking, talking, shaving, or brush-
ing his teeth brought on the painful paroxysms. He had lost forty
pounds in weight. There was a partial anesthesia over the entire
maxillary and mandibular divisions of the fifth nerve but, in spite of
this marked diminution in sensitivity, even the lightest touch to
certain parts of his face would initiate a severe attack. Attacks could
be set off by contact near the nasal ala, within the margin of the
nostril, near the outer margin of the lip, near the canthus of the eye,
and at two areas in the gum on each side of his two remaining
incisor teeth in the right upper jaw. Each of these sensitive points
was injected several times in the course of a three weeks' treatment.
Whenever he had a twinge of pain, the site from which the pain
seemed to originate was infiltrated with novocaine. The attacks
rapidly diminished in frequency and severity. There was a temporary exacerbation when the two incisor teeth were removed. He
remained entirely free from pain from June until December. Then
he had a mild recurrence requiring five injections to control. In
March, 1942, sharp paroxysms began again. They were relieved
within two weeks by a few injections and the fitting of an upper
plate.

These four cases represent the favorable response to local
treatment by novocaine injections. Considered alone they
would be misleading because it is only in selected cases that
the method is successful. However, it succeeds in a sufficiently
large number of cases to justify its being tried before more
radical methods of treatment are undertaken. Its interest here
lies in the fact that a temporarily acting anesthetic solution
sometimes abolishes pain syndromes of long standing. The
first treatment rarely accomplishes more than a very short alleviation of pain, and when the local effect wears off the pain
may be increased. This seems to be as true of the cases that
eventually yield to treatment as of those that do not. I do not

know why this should be so, unless it is that the local injury caused by the needle gives rise to additional afferent impulses acting on an already hypersensitized receiving center in the brain. In the favorable case the primary exacerbation of symptoms is followed by a period of relative relief, which tends to grow longer as treatment progresses. Secondary trigger zones disappear, the sensitiveness of the face diminishes, the paroxysms of pain become less intense and farther apart, reflex disturbances and paresthesias fade, and the pain ceases. It is as if the thalamus or some other brain center was gradually undergoing some change that tended to raise toward normal an abnormally low pain threshold.

## CHAPTER X

## Phantom Limb Pain

The term "phantom limb" is used to designate the illusion of the persistent presence of a limb after it has been amputated. It is a remarkable fact that the great majority of patients who have had a limb removed will retain, long after the stump has healed, perhaps for the remainder of their lives, a vivid sense of the presence of the absent member. Often the vivid quality of the sensory illusion causes the patient to be more aware of the phantom than of the normal limb. Sometimes the sensations are distressing and occasionally there is a degree of pain that so preoccupies the patient as to destroy his social usefulness.

The phenomenon of the phantom limb is much more common than is generally realized. Mitchell [85] states that he found it in 86 of 90 patients he personally examined. Leriche [64] believes it occurs in 98 per cent of all cases of major limb amputations. It is quite possible that the physician who is sought out by those suffering from phantom limb pain may get an erroneous impression of its frequency and of the severity of the symptoms. On the other hand, any casual questioning of patients who have had amputations is likely to give an equally distorted impression, because many of these are reluctant to talk about experiences which they have learned are regarded by layman and physician alike as being of purely psychic origin. I have been frequently rebuffed in an attempt to elicit a history of phantom limb sensations. Not infrequently I have been told that no phantom phenomena exist, and only at a later date have been told the real story. An attorney of my acquaintance, who had had his right hand amputated just above the wrist some thirty years previously, vigorously denied any phantom sensations in the hand and pounded the stump on the table to demonstrate its lack of sensitiveness. But, when convinced of my sincere interest in the phenomena, he admitted that ever since his amputation it had felt to him that the tip of his index finger had been pressing into the side of the distal phalanx of the thumb.

My experience, based on an examination of a considerable number of amputations at the Oregon State Industrial Accident Commission, would give me the impression similar to that expressed by Mitchell and Leriche, that the sensation of a phantom limb was almost universal and would also lead me to believe that a large percentage of such cases suffered from distressing and painful sensations. However, this impression has been modified by questioning many casually encountered cases of amputation. I have talked with a few individuals with lower limb amputations, who apparently have lost all consciousness of the lost member, but I can only recall one case of upper limb amputation in which the entire extremity was "completely gone." This man stated that he had had mild phantom limb pain for two years after his amputation, after which all sensations disappeared.

In cases of high amputation, almost never is the complete extremity felt to be present. In the upper arm amputation, for instance, the patient is usually conscious of the fingers and hand, occasionally of the wrist, rarely of the elbow, and almost never of the forearm, or of the portion of the arm between the end of the stump and the phantom elbow. There are exceptions to this and a patient may complain of such bizarre symptoms as itching in the cubital fossa or a sensation of burning irritation as if the dorsum of the forearm had been denuded of skin. Occasionally the elbow is not actually felt but the patient deduces its position by the location of the phantom hand. Frequently the arm seems to be shortened, in rare instances to the degree that the hand seems to be attached directly to the stump. Although there is frequently a foreshortening of the intervening arm, the hand is usually said to be of normal size. It is remarkable how accurately these individuals can describe the exact posture of the phantom limb. More remarkable still is the retention of the ability to move the phantom digits, that is occasionally observed. Free voluntary movements of the fingers are quite exceptional, but occasionally one encounters an individual who can move his hand and fingers in any way he wishes. When asked to perform movements, such a patient will say, "Now my hand is open, now it is closed, now I am touching my thumb with each finger in turn, etc." When the amputation has been performed at the wrist level, voluntary movements of the phantom fingers are accompanied by appropriate contractions of the forearm muscles, but the patient with an upper arm amputation will state with equal assurance that he is carrying out identical movements, even though there is no outward evidence to support his statement. The remarkable feature of this assurance in describing changes in posture becomes apparent when one recalls that these individuals have no proprioceptive end-organs in the muscles, tendons, and joints that are felt as if being voluntarily moved. Mitchell [85] (p. 358), in commenting on voluntary movements of phantom limb, says: "The physiology of the day accepts the belief that all of our accurate notions as to the amount of power put forth, and as to the parts thus stirred, reach the sensorium from the muscles acted on and the parts moved. It would appear, however, from the statements here made, as if coevally with the willing of a motion, there came to consciousness, perhaps from the spinal ganglia acted upon, some information as to these points. If, in reply to this, I be told that the constancy of long habit may have associated memorially with certain ganglionic activities the ideas of local movements, I should hardly feel that this was an answer, because in some of my cases the amputations took place so early in life that there was no remembrance of the lost limb, and yet, twenty years after, a volition directed to the hand seemed to cause movement, which appeared to be as capable of definite regulation, and was as plainly felt to occur as if it had been the other arm which was moved. Probably, then, a part of those ideas which we are presumed to obtain through the muscular sense are really coincident with, and instituted by, the originative act of will, or else are messages sent to the sensorium from the spinal ganglia which every act of motor volition incites."

This is a most interesting observation. It is somewhat difficult to accept at its face value because more often than not the phantom hand occupies a fixed posture from which no effort of the will is capable of moving it.

The sensation of a fixed and tense posture involving the phantom fingers or toes is extremely common. It is probably the basis for such statements as: "The doctor forgot to straighten out my fingers before he took my arm off," and the folk-lore that deals with the digging up of amputated extremities to change the posture of digits or remove some irritating foreign material. The sense of tension seems to vary. In some, it is mildly annoying and at times can be disregarded. In others it seems to be almost unbearable. Occasionally there occur involuntary changes in position and the fingers become pressed against one another in a new posture or cramp from which the subject is unable to release them. Occasionally the fingers or their nails may seem to be cutting into the palm, the nails being pulled off, or there is a sensation of boring up through the bones of the fingers into the hand. There are other types of pain felt in the phantom extremity that have been described as tearing, pressing, and stabbing, but the commonest pain and the one that is usually most persistent is that of a burning sense of heat as if the hand were held too close to a fire.

All of these sensations ascribed to the phantom limb are found to vary not only from case to case but from day to day in the same individual. Any irritation of the stump, such as a light blow or the wearing of an artificial limb, may change a mildly annoying group of symptoms to an unbearable torture. Nervousness, worry, and fatigue seem to be capable of altering the severity of the sensations. Exposure of the stump to cold very frequently aggravates the symptoms and a considerable number complain that changes in the weather affect their condition. In some, a change from clear to rainy weather seems to increase their pain as much as does actual exposure to cold.

In describing the phantom limb syndrome thus far I have omitted all mention of the stump. This omission was purposeful because, in my experience, although abnormalities of the stump are often associated with sensations ascribed to the phantom limb, the two conditions do not seem to be interdependent. At least it is certain that the "sensory ghost" can exist in the presence of a perfectly constructed, and insensitive stump. When pain forms an important feature in the sensations, it is much more common to find associated changes in the stump. The commonest objective sign observed in the stump in association with severe phantom limb pain, is that of coldness. The temperature of the stump may be as much as 10° C. colder than the same level on the normal extremity. Excessive sweating and hyperesthesia are also frequent concomitants of the pain. The stump may be clammy with sweat, and many patients assert that they sweat much more from the axilla of the amputated side than from the normal side. The entire stump may be hyperesthetic, but more often the sensitiveness is limited to certain areas, such as parts of the operative scar. When such superficially hyperesthetic spots are lightly stimulated the patient may experience sharp pains in the phantom hand, or the entire pain picture may be aggravated. K. E. Livingston [72] reports one remarkable instance of a sensitive point in the scar of a thigh amputation, in which an injection of a few minims of novocaine solution not only alleviated the pain, but was followed by a prompt relaxation of the muscles in the stump, and a subjective sensation as if the phantom limb could now be moved from the abnormal and tense posture in which it had been held since the amputation.

One of the most interesting phenomena observed in stumps is the abnormal activity of the muscles. Very often there are fibrillary twitchings of small muscle bundles, and at times the stump jerks spasmodically and involuntarily. One patient told me that when he attended a baseball game he had to constantly hold the stump clamped against his side with his other hand; otherwise, in moments of excitement it was liable to flip up unexpectedly and strike his neighbor. In other patients the stump has periods of sustained clonic contractions. These attacks of uncontrollable jerking may be associated with a particularly severe bout of pain, but occasionally a stump is seen which is in constant motion. In discussing these clonic contractions, which he calls "choreiform movements," Mitchell [85] says (p. 347): "While emotion may cause involuntary movement, it may also check chorciform spasms, as in the case of Colonel Parr, whose arm-stump was never in repose a moment, except when, at Cedar Mountain, his regiment being cut off for a time, and in danger of being taken,—the restless limb was seen for some hours to hang motionless at his side."

## TREATMENT

No single method of treatment has been found that will give uniformly satisfactory results in the relief of phantom limb pain. The surgeon who encounters an occasional instance of this syndrome usually focuses his attention on the stump. He is aware of the blind effort of nerve fibers to continue growing, long after an amputation has taken place, and he assumes that if the pain symptoms have reality, they must arise as a result of stimulation of the cut fibers. He may visualize the growing fibers as being compressed in scar tissue, or stimulated in some way by the local ischemia of the stump. He is likely to feel that this opinion is confirmed if he finds a palpable neuroma that is sensitive to pressure, and particularly if the patient tells him that pressure over the nerve trunk at a higher level tends to relieve the pain temporarily. He therefore undertakes a remodeling of the stump, and excision of neuromas, or an amputation at a higher level with every expectation of relieving the patient. In a few instances this expectation proves to be justified by the outcome, but in the great majority of cases the relief, if obtained at all, is limited to a few weeks or months, and then the whole syndrome recurs. When the pain returns there is almost always a return of the coldness, hyperesthesia and excessive sweating. This is the case, even when reamputation is done high above the former level, and in tissues that had not previously been cold or hyperesthetic.

Molotkoff [86] believes that the pain is due to constant irritation of cutaneous nerves, rather than any activity in the larger
palpable neuromas, and he advises the division of several nerves
at the same operation. Leriche [64] has also advised section of
several nerves at the same time and has advocated dividing the
nerve trunks well above the neuromas, and then doing an
immediate end-to-end suture of the cut ends. More recently
Leriche has concluded that all peripheral operations are too
likely to fail, and in their place has advocated measures that
block the sympathetic nerve impulses. He reports a number of
favorable results from the infiltration of sympathetic ganglia
with novocaine solution, and says that although a single injection may not confer lasting relief, repeated injections may
bring about a cure. In upper limb amputations he infiltrates
the stellate ganglion and sometimes the second thoracic. My
own observations [77] confirm those reported by Leriche, but
my injections have usually been done at a lower thoracic level.
I have found that novocaine injections as low as the sixth and
seventh thoracic ganglia can exert a favorable influence on an
upper limb stump and on the phantom limb pain.

CASE No. 19.—Mr. R. H. D., a man aged 54, lost his right hand
on October 31, 1933. He was employed in a shingle mill and became
caught in a saw which severed the right forearm in its middle third
and slashed a great wound in his chest and abdomen. At the end
of nine weeks his wounds were completely healed, but there was
restriction in the range of motion at the shoulder. He also began to
complain of pain and sensitiveness in the stump and of increasing
tension in the phantom hand. The arm and shoulder muscles began
a convulsive jerking which was annoying and uncontrollable. This
was associated with "cramping" in the fingers. He said it felt as if
there were a wire down the center of his arm to which his fingers
were attached. He also spoke of feeling as though some force were

pulling on the wire "as if to pull the fingers up through the arm." At times the hand felt hot, as if held by force too close to a hot stove, and the fingers became the seat of intolerable burning. He could not move the fingers voluntarily, but they tended to shift their position over one another, and in so doing would "get caught in cramps." The thumb was apt to abduct and then slowly draw down over the fingers with great force; then the wrist would slowly flex strongly, and the whole hand and wrist would ache. Interspersed between the muscular contractions he felt knife-like stabs of pain through the hand and fingers. When the burning sensation was absent, the general feeling of the hand and wrist was one of coldness, although this was seldom of an unpleasant degree.

As the patient's symptoms progressed he was noted to have a rapid pulse, to tremble all over and to sweat profusely while talking to the examiner. His physical and mental attitude showed a shrinking away from all contacts, and he was incapable of carrying out the simplest transactions. He could not read for any length of time, and his sleep was disturbed. Hyperesthesia of the stump prevented him from wearing his artificial limb. The jerking of his muscles, his mental attitude and what was considered an exaggerated hyperesthesia of the stump led to his being classed as a case of "hysteria." He repeatedly refused to consider a closure of his claim against the State Industrial Accident Commission, claiming that his pain prevented him from ever doing any work again. A long course of physical therapy, excision of numerous "neuromas," correction of dental sepsis, and psychotherapy failed to bring about the slightest improvement in his condition.

In June, 1935, a 2 per cent solution of novocaine was injected near the third, fourth and fifth thoracic sympathetic ganglions on the affected side. A small amount of iodized poppy-seed oil was injected through each needle before it was withdrawn, and subsequent roentgenograms showed the material deposited along the sides of the vertebral bodies near the ribs from the third to the sixth. There was no Horner syndrome, but there was a prompt subjective sense of warmth and relaxation in the fingers of the phantom hand. The thumb slowly moved outward from the fist position, and one by one the fingers opened. The stabbing pains and the jerking of the stump ceased. The two neuromas which had been marked out on the stump before the injection were no longer sensitive.

Examined in November, the patient was found to be wearing his artificial limb continuously. He said he occasionally felt sensations of cold or transient pains in the phantom hand and that at rare intervals the shoulder muscles would jerk, but he expressed himself as delighted with the improvement in his condition. The hyperesthesia of the stump was gone; he slept soundly at night; he had gained in weight; and the change in his physical condition and mental attitude was apparent in his demeanor and in his request for a closure of his claim. He reported to me a year later to show me a device that he had made to improve the function of his artificial hand, and at that time stated that there had been no recurrence of pain.

This case and the one described in the first chapter represent the most favorable outcome from this method of treatment. More often than not the method fails to accomplish a permanent cure. The following case record illustrates the type classified as "unsatisfactory" result.

Case No. 20.—Mr. C. H., a man aged 60, had his right arm partially avulsed at the shoulder when it became caught in a gear in November, 1931. The amputation was completed within a few hours, and a large denuded area in the axilla was partially covered with grafts of skin from the abdomen. He was not particularly conscious of the phantom hand during the first six weeks after the amputation. He then began to have three different types of pain ascribed to the absent limb. The first sensation was a continuous burning heat, "like fire in the fingers and hand." The index finger was least affected; the thumb and remaining three fingers were most affected. The second sensation was that of "tightness" associated with a sense of "trembling, drawing and twisting" in the hand and arm. The third type of pain was intermittent and was described as "shooting stabs of pain" throughout the limb. These pains were variable in intensity, but he claimed never to have been free from them for more than twenty minutes during his waking hours. He did not think that his sleep was seriously disturbed and stated that the arm "goes off to sleep two or three times before I can get to sleep." He wore a steel-reënforced leather shield over the shoulder to protect it from any contact, the scar being so sensitive that blowing one's breath across it caused him to cringe and the shoulder muscles to jerk.

At the time of the injection in October, 1935, the phantom hand was described as being in a claw-like position, which he could not alter except to move the index finger slightly. This patient knew that some sort of test was to be performed on his back, but I had purposely refrained from explaining the procedure or telling him what he might expect from it. Novocaine was injected near the thoracic sympathetic ganglions from the third to the sixth, and he was asked to report any changes in sensation. He promptly reported that the hand was becoming warm and that he could move all of his fingers. There was a pleasant sense of relaxation, and the "twisting" tension disappeared. The scar was no longer hyperesthetic, and the jerking of the muscles subsided. In the next few days the phantom hand, which had always felt somewhat smaller than normal, seemed to shrink still more, so that the arm felt to be "about six inches long" and the hand "about as big as a dollar." Examined three months after the injection, he reported a satisfactory degree of relief, but fourteen months later he returned, complaining of a recurrence of the original pain. On the day he was brought to me by his local physician he had a sharp stab of pain, so severe that he fell to the floor in a faint. On December 14, 1936, a 2 per cent solution of novocaine was injected near the third to the seventh thoracic sympathetic ganglia and was followed by the injection of a small amount of dilute solution of quinine and ethyl carbamate (urethane).

He again reported a prompt relief from pain and tension, but by March, 1937, the fingers no longer felt movable, although the pain had not recurred. The dorsum of the hand was said to feel colder than the palm. In May he reported that the pain had come back. A thoracic ganglionectomy was performed by the posterior approach, the fourth and fifth sympathetic ganglions being excised. Again there was relief from the pain, but within a month it had begun to come back. In August I injected novocaine near the stellate ganglion, without appreciably altering his subjective complaints, and later in the same month I divided the brachial plexus high in his neck. The nerve trunks were divided close to the vertebral foramina, alcohol was injected, and the cut ends were closed with fine silk sutures. I regret that I cannot say definitely whether or not the division of the nerve trunks was proximal or distal to the point at which the gray rami join them. The nerve trunks at the point of section were not involved in scar tissue and appeared normal in cross section. Instead of relieving his pain, the operation made it worse. He said that the hand was as tense as ever and the pain unbearable. He entered the hospital in December, 1937, prepared for a chordotomy, but he wished me to first try more novocaine injections. An infiltration of the upper thoracic ganglia with this solution relaxed and warmed the hand. The pain was again relieved for a few weeks. This man has reported from time to time for further injections which alleviate his pain for a while, but the case must be classified as an "unsatisfactory" result. It is of considerable interest to note that an injection of the sixth and seventh thoracic ganglia, carried out seven months after resection of the fourth and fifth, gave him relief for a time, implying that during this interval there had been regeneration of the fibers across the gap created by the operation.

Bailey and Moersch [5] in a valuable analysis of 105 cases of amputations, are convinced that the symptoms cannot be ascribed to peripheral irritation. They state: "That the problem is more than one of irritation of peripheral nerves in scar tissue, or of dilated or constricted blood vessels either locally or in the arachnoid meninges, seems by now to have passed from the stage of supposition to a foregone conclusion." Their summary concludes: "The mechanism of the pain is not clear, and at present we hesitate to accept the theory of ascending neuritis or peripheral irritation. It seems more likely that its origin is central (that is, intracranial) and most probably psychic. Some of the evidence in our cases suggests the possibility that it is some form of obsession neurosis."

This interpretation of the phantom limb phenomena apparently represents a majority opinion. It is pointed out that if the syndrome arose as a result of peripheral irritation, the excision of neuromata or a re-amputation should cure it. Often these procedures fail, and any relief they confer is limited to a few weeks or months. Pressure on a nerve trunk may alleviate the pain for a time, yet cutting that nerve rarely affords lasting benefit. Even extensive rhizotomies may fail to cure the pain. All of these observations are used as arguments against the existence of peripheral irritants as a cause for the phantom limb phenomena.

In favor of a central origin, and the view that the symptoms must be an obsession neurosis, other observations have been emphasized. There are no peripheral end-organs to account for the sensory impressions of posture, touch, movement and the like; the patient usually feels most vividly the parts of the limb that have the greatest representation in the cortex (i.e., the hand, index finger, etc.); the fixed posture of the phantom, is commonly reported to be that in which the injured limb was last seen by the patient; and, finally, the evidences of nervousness and emotional instability which may be evident by the time the patient comes under observation in his quest for medical assistance, are said to indicate a temperament that favors the development of an obsession neurosis.

As clinical observations no one could object to any of these statements, but used as arguments to rule out the possibility that peripheral irritation can have any part in the syndrome, and to prove the purely psychic origin of the condition, they are inconclusive. As I have already intimated, my own observations point toward exactly opposite conclusions, i.e., that peripheral irritation, while by no means constituting the whole story, *is* an important factor in the phantom limb pain syndrome, and that the symptoms *are not* purely psychic in origin. Of thirty-six cases I have personally studied, three have been cured, and a number of others have been considerably benefited, by operations confined to the stump. I have carried out novocaine injections of the sympathetic ganglia on more than thirty of these cases, and although only nine of these can be classified as satisfactory results in respect to permanency, more than two-thirds of this series experienced changes in their symptoms as a result of the injection and were relieved of pain for variable periods of time. The subjective alterations in sensation that follow novocaine injection are of considerable scientific interest and the similarity in these changes as they are reported by case after case, has furnished what, to me, seems to be convincing evidence that the symptoms are not psychic in origin.

Under the immediate influence of the injection the stump becomes warm and dry, and at the same time the phantom extremity is felt to grow warm and relaxed. The pain disappears, the cramped posture is released, and one by one the phantom fingers open and can be voluntarily moved. The patient may know nothing of the nature or the purpose of the injection, he may never have heard of a similar case, he has no reason to expect that the injection made at a considerable distance from the stump will affect his long-established complaints, and yet he will report exactly the same train of subjective alterations in the phantom. In January, 1939, an orthopedic surgeon asked me to inject one of his cases. I suggested that this surgeon make the injection himself without telling the patient anything more than that a test of some kind was being done, and I purposely did not examine the patient or talk to him before the test was carried out. The sequence of events that I had observed in my own patients was reported by this surgeon as taking place during the injection, and the phantom hand, which had been immovable for years, relaxed and the fingers felt as if they could be moved voluntarily. Incidentally, the pain did not recur when the novocaine effects disappeared, and the benefit seems to have been permanent.

It is difficult for me to make these observations consistent with an "obsession neurosis." The fixed posture of the phantom previous to the injection might suggest an obsession, but to have it change so abruptly after the injection, to the surprise of the subject, and exactly like the changes reported by other patients suggests to me that some physiologic change has taken place to modify the central perceptions. There are other observations that argue against an obsession or fixed idea, some of which are illustrated by a case I injected three years ago. The patient was a young man whose hand and arm had been dragged into a hot paper press. About ten days elapsed between the time of the accident and the amputation of the arm. In that interval he saw the hand and arm every time they were dressed. The hand was spread out flat on the moist dressings. Yet he claims that from the moment he recovered from his anesthetic after the amputation, the hand felt to him as if it were drawn into a tense claw position. It did not change from this position for two years, and no voluntary movement was possible until his injection. Novocaine was infiltrated into the region of the fourth, fifth and sixth thoracic sympathetic ganglia of the affected side. Nothing was done to the stump. Under the influence of the novocaine the stump warmed, the claw posture relaxed and the fingers could be moved voluntarily. The hand remained relaxed and movable for only a few days and then gradually returned to the claw position. There was no return of pain at this time, and the sense of tension was mild in degree. A second injection permitted the fingers to open again and this time they remained open.

Dramatic as these reported changes in the phantom limb may be, they are not convincing evidence because they are dependent upon subjective sensations. It is conceivable that suggestion therapy might modify the obsession so that the patient became convinced that some change was taking place in the sensory ghost of his absent limb. But there are objective evidences that an actual change has taken place in the stump. A stump that was cold, hyperesthetic and clammy with sweat, becomes warm, dry and insensitive under the influence of the novocaine injection. Tender neuromas or scars may lose their tenderness. These alterations, coming immediately after the injection might have been anticipated. But the observation that has impressed me most is that in the cases in which the pain does not recur, *the coldness, hyperesthesia and excessive sweating do not recur*. In the phantom limb syndrome described in the "Introduction" the temperature of the stump was more than 10° C. colder than the other arm five days before his injection in October, 1934. Five years after this injection the temperature of the stump was within two degrees of the other side, and the excessive sweating and tenderness had not recurred.

Riddoch,[102] in a comprehensive discussion of "Phantom

Limbs and Body Shape," expresses the conviction that the phantom limb phenomena are real, in the sense that they depend upon the stimulation of the cut ends of nerves in the stump. He thinks that the impulses evoked by this peripheral stimulation register as sensations which act to maintain the integrity of the "plastic model" of self, and in terms of the model, are "projected and interpreted as if the limb were still present." He believes that when a limb is lost, the incoming impulses from the stump are immediately subjected to central inhibition, and that when the peripheral stimulation is moderate in degree, the central inhibition may eventually lead to a shrinkage and final disappearance of the phantom limb. But when the peripheral stimulation is intense, the pain sensations overcome central inhibition and the painful phantom may persist indefinitely. He says: "Massive painful stimulation from abnormalities in the stump is always able to overcome central inhibition and the phantom remains for so long as pain is referred to it. When psycho-physiological inhibition, and so adaptability, is subnormal, even a painless phantom part may last indefinitely; and, on the other hand, inhibition may be temporarily reduced by ill-health or emotional disturbance with the resultant re-appearance of the phantom that had gone. Thus, the two forces, excitation and inhibition are in continual interaction in the attempt to establish a new body shape. . . .

"In conclusion, contemplation of the story of the phantom limb forces the realization of the striking contrast presented by the difficulty which the individual has in accepting, physiologically as well as psychologically, his shortened limb, and his possession of a strong natural aptitude to elongate his limbs in the use of tools. When, for example, he is (after amputation) wearing his artificial limb he feels with its foot and can distinguish between irregularities on the ground. There is no essential difference between this achievement and that of the surgeon who projects his fingers to the end of his probe, or that of the edentulous who incorporates his artificial teeth. In the same way, the trained motorist identifies his car with himself, the airman with his machine, and the angler with his fly at the end of a long line. Samuel Butler, who developed this idea, called tools detachable limbs and maintained that the capacity to employ them in this way is one of the main characteristics which distinguishes man from lower animals. The competency of this attitude for projection varies in different individuals for reasons that are inborn, as well as of training. But, strong as it is, it is at once inhibited if discomfort or pain is evoked by contact of the tool with the body. The dental plate or artificial limb is immediately rejected as a foreign body if there is an ulcer on the gum or a tender neuroma at the end of a stump. It is another illustration of the dominance of pain over adaptive functions."

I like these interpretations of Riddoch's. His use of Head's concept of "body schemes" and his insistence on the existence of peripheral irritation in the stump to maintain the syndrome of the phantom limb are in accord with my view. I would add one other feature that seems to be necessary to complete a reasonable interpretation of the reported observations. There must be a third agency interposed between the peripheral sources of irritation and the plastic model of self. It is a physiologic agency that I think of as being in the spinal cord, on which the original irritants act to bring about the abnormal state of the blood vessels and sweat glands, the cutaneous hyperesthesia and the changes involving the skeletal muscles. In my opinion the internuncial pool may be the agency which acquires a momentum that may obviate a cure by reamputation or excision of neuromata; it may be the agency which is acted upon by the sympathetic injections; and it may be through this agency that a normal physiologic status is restored.

## CHAPTER XI

# *Technic*

I do not wish to emphasize technic. The details of the various surgical operations for periarterial sympathectomy, ganglionectomy, and novocaine injection of the ganglionic chain are amply described elsewhere. What little there is to be said about the technic of trigger point injection and the method I now employ for permanently closing the end of a cut nerve, is mentioned in anticipation of questions that might be asked in regard to procedure as it relates to pain interpretation.

The first question that might be asked is, why is novocaine solution used in preference to other solutions? It is used in the majority of cases, because, in my hands, this solution has given better results than any other preparation I have tried. In addition it is cheap, convenient and its pharmacologic properties are well known. In a number of instances I have tried injecting salt solution, and sometimes, as in expanding a small neuroma or a sensitive scar, it has given good results. It is more painful to the patient and it fails to afford relief from pain much more often than it succeeds. When it succeeds I am inclined to attribute the result to the mechanical action of the fluid as it distends scar tissue, combined perhaps, with the local inflammatory reaction produced by any injection. Even needle punctures, such as are sometimes employed in the treatment of a subdeltoid bursitis, may seem to hasten the curative process.

There is a drug on the market under the trade name of "Sarapin" with which I have secured favorable results. It is said to be prepared from an extract of the pitcher-plant, whose flower catches and paralyzes flying insects. The drug is said to produce a selective blockade of conduction in the small fibers of the C group, without materially reducing conduction in the large fibers of the A group. Theoretically, there should be definite advantages in the use of a drug that might thus be expected to relieve the disagreeable type of pain without abolishing touch sensibility. I have used sarapin in a number of cases of chronic back disability with good results. My impression has been, however, that these results are no better, if as good, as those obtained by the use of novocaine solution. I have tried another proprietary drug known as "Aciform 2" for which remarkable therapeutic powers are claimed. This preparation causes a momentary stinging pain at the site of injection, followed in many instances by relief of pain. The solution is said to contain 0.0018 gm. of formic acid; 0.0002 gm. sulphur; 0.004 gm. iodine; 0.0001 cc. terpene (from camphor); 0.055 cc. of 95 per cent alcohol and water q.s. to make one cubic centimeter. It might be anticipated that such a combination would set up considerable local reaction, but in the small quantities which are used it seems to have no unpleasant after-effects, and possibly the local reaction may contribute to the beneficial result. It has been recommended particularly for arthritis, a condition which I have had little occasion to treat. In the treatment of sensitive spots, which I have called "trigger points," but which may represent a local fascitis or myositis, it has given a number of favorable results. Again, however, as with sarapin, I have not been able to convince myself that the results are better than with novocaine solution. I still employ one or the other of these preparations from time to time when my patient has, or thinks he has, a real sensitiveness to novocaine.

A question that is certain to be asked is: How may the trigger point be identified? In general this might be answered by saying that its sensitiveness identifies it. But this is not an adequate answer because in the well-developed case the sensitiveness may be very widespread. What the patient can tell of the nature and site of the original injury is often of assistance in finding it. The fact that the whole syndrome developed as a result of this local injury suggests that here may be found the trigger mechanism which maintains it. During the examination of the patient, a back injury say, the palpation proceeds toward the spots he has indicated as representing the most sensitive zones, or the site from which the pain seems to spring. Once a suspected point has been marked out on the skin, the palpation is varied, so that the patient is required to repeatedly assist in identifying this particular spot. A variation in the location of the spot, or uncertainty as to its repeated identification, suggests that this may not be the true trigger point. Finally, the results of injection are of aid in identifying the trigger point, because in many instances, secondary points of tenderness tend to disappear spontaneously when the sensitiveness of the offending focus has been abolished.

The needle is used as a probe in finding the trigger point. I use as fine needles as I can get, usually a 2-inch needle of No. 26 or No. 27 caliber. The needle is introduced in the same direction that pressure was exerted to elicit the tenderness, and it is pushed forward until it encounters tissue that resists its passage or that seems to be abnormally sensitive. The novocaine solution is injected under sufficient pressure to expand the resistant tissue. The quantity injected is small, usually 5 cc. or less. If during this injection the pain is reproduced or exaggerated, and in particular, if its typical reference is experienced, the evidence suggests that this particular spot may represent a trigger point. The real test, however, is the reaction that is obtained after the injection. Sometimes, the relief of pain and the release of muscle spasm that immediately follows the injection is spectacular. For a few hours the patient may be convinced that he is cured, or at least well on the road to recovery. In rare instances this immediate reaction persists indefinitely, but more often it is followed by a recurrence of symptoms, frequently in an exaggerated degree.

An aggravation of symptoms for many hours after the local anesthetic effect has worn off, is very often the factor which leads to the abandonment of the injection treatments. The patient asserts in no uncertain terms that he is through with this form of therapy. A few years ago, I would have agreed with him that the method had been tried and had failed, but on the basis of a wider experience, I have come to feel that the temporary exacerbation of symptoms may actually be a favorable sign. I have the feeling that I am treading close to a hypersensitized zone possessed of dynamic potentialities. And I try to let my patient understand that I do not consider his reaction an unfavorable one. Usually he consents to try one more injection, and fortunately, subsequent reactions are so much less, or the secondary periods of relief that follow it are so encouraging to both the patient and the surgeon that treatment can be carried on until it is evident that it is useful or is not. The type of case which, to me, seems most unpromising is the one that is never certain of the location of a trigger point, and never experiences the secondary period of improvement. My experience would indicate that this type probably will not respond favorably to any number of injections, and that after a very few trials some other method of treatment should be substituted for the injections.

The question might be asked as to how the surgeon may lessen the chances of the development of trigger points in the

scar tissue left by an operation? The general answer to this lies
in following the cardinal principles of good surgery in the gen-
tleness and respect accorded to the tissues. But that this is not
a complete answer is demonstrated by the fact that sensitive
scars may occur after the most careful handling of the tissues.
The most superficial of wounds, such as former generations of
physicians used in the practice of "bleeding," not infrequently
were followed by "bent arm" or other serious consequences
suggestive of the causalgic states. Just as thousands of such
minor wounds were made by surgeons or barbers without producing a trigger point, so it happens that the surgeon of today
can cut and manipulate tissues with a certain large degree of
immunity from serious after-effects. Perhaps his respectful handling of tissue will reduce the hazard of trigger point formation, yet I do not feel that it altogether eliminates the danger.
As I have said elsewhere, it is possible that the development of
a causalgic state may be a function of the temperament of an
individual patient, but more probably it represents a happen-
stance, in which just the right combination of factors, perhaps
scar imprisoning sensory filaments, takes place to create a focus
of sustained irritation.

What can be done to prevent the formation of neuromas?
So far as I know, nothing. I have tried most of the accepted
methods purporting to prevent neuroma formation, and believe
that they all fail of this purpose. For many years I routinely
used alcohol injection of cut nerves in my amputations and in
reamputating for painful stumps, but I am convinced that this
neither prevents neuroma formation nor lessens materially the
chances that the subsequent neuroma will be painful. In fact,
I have wondered whether the use of this irritating and sclerotic
drug may not actually enhance the possibility of the development of distressing postoperative symptoms. In resecting a neu-

roma in an amputation stump my present method for closing cut nerve ends has for its purpose the avoidance of three factors, which I feel might act to cause pain, (1) the use of irritant chemicals; (2) the contact of growing nerve fibers with nonneural tissue; and (3) the involvement of the nerve stump in the operative scar.

The nerve is drawn down into the wound as far as its elasticity will permit, using firm, steady traction. In the uppermost exposed segment, novocaine is injected so as to distend about an inch of the trunk. Through the center of the distended segment a traction suture of chromic gut is placed. Just below the segment a circular incision is made through the nerve sheath and a cuff of sheath is rolled upward to a point close to the traction suture. The nerve is cut transversely below the cuff, the nerve stump now being held down into the wound by the traction suture. With mosquito clips on the margins of the cuff, it is brought down over the nerve stump and the clips twisted so that the cuff snugly encases the cut end. A ligature is tied firmly around the puckered twist of empty cuff below the nerve end. Then, just above the traction suture, and still within the segment that has been distended with novocaine, a physiologic interruption * of nerve continuity is carried out. This is accomplished by crushing the nerve fibers with a forceps, in such a manner that fiber continuity is broken, without severing the nerve sheath. The traction suture is then cut and the nerve stump retracts out of the wound.

The purpose of the physiologic division of the nerve well above the cut end is to permit time for firm healing of the cuff

---

* This use of the term "physiologic interruption" is not exact. It is used more correctly to apply to a temporary blockade of nerve impulses by anesthetic drugs or pressure. However, the method approximates a physiologic interruption in the sense that the intraneural pattern is not seriously disturbed and the nerve sheath remains intact.

# Suggested Method for Permanent Closure of Large Nerve Trunks

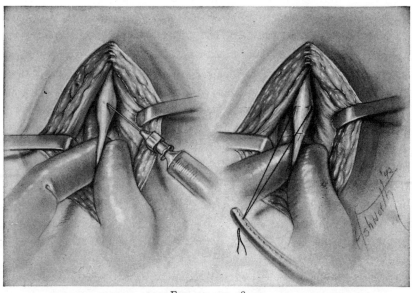

Figs. 17 and 18

The nerve trunk is distended with novocaine.

Traction suture placed. Circular incision in sheath.

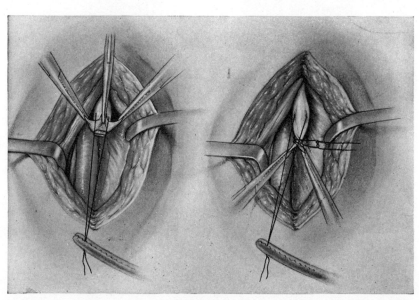

Figs. 19 and 20

Cuff of sheath is dissected upward, and trunk divided.

Cuff of sheath is pulled down over nerve stump, twisted and ligated.

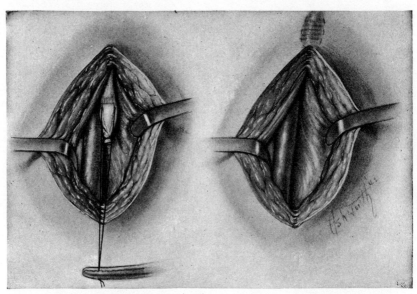

FIGS. 21 AND 22

The nerve is crushed with forceps above traction suture.

Traction suture is cut and nerve stump retracts out of the wound.

of sheath over the nerve stump before growing fibers reach this level. It is hoped thereby to lessen the chances for nerve fibers to escape from the sheath to make contact with non-neural tissues, as they almost inevitably seem to do in "trap-door" closures, and other methods I have tried. I do not expect this method to prevent neuroma formation, and I have not used it for a long enough period or in enough cases to know that it will reduce the chances of the neuroma being sensitive or the source of phantom pain. This whole subject of the treatment of cut nerve ends deserves further investigation.

Section Three

# INTERPRETATIONS

## CHAPTER XII

*Protopathic Pain*

The final section of this monograph has been difficult to write. I have felt overwhelmed by the enormous accumulation of data bearing on pain interpretation, by the many controversial subjects that are so intimately interrelated, and by my own inability to answer so many questions. I have been tempted to avoid the task of interpretation, by simply presenting my clinical observations and letting the reader make whatever deductions he could from them. If this had been the plan I would have added many more case reports, because it is the impact of case after case, all of them presenting similar features, that convinces the observer of the reality of each clinical syndrome. I would have discussed the scalenus anticus syndrome, meralgia paresthetica, traumatic osteoporosis and many other clinical entities which I believe are related to the cases which have been presented.

But I am not primarily concerned with convincing the reader of the reality of particular syndromes, nor with advocating any special method for treating them. My purpose has been to present a concept of pain, and an interpretation of its possible mechanisms that more and more tends to influence my approach to clinical problems. My interpretations have been influenced by the ideas of many men. I find that I cannot even say with assurance from what particular sources my present groping interpretations have come. There are a few studies, however, that have had a profound influence on my thinking. Two of these concern "protopathic" pain, and "hyperalgesia."

### PROTOPATHIC PAIN

It is well known that disturbances of sensory experience occur after the anatomic interruption of sensory nerves. Sensations elicited by innocuous stimuli may be peculiarly unpleasant. There are two occasions when this phenomenon is most apparent. One occurs immediately after the nerve section, when it can be shown that stimulation of an "intermediate zone" between the completely anesthetic area and the normally innervated skin, may result in perverted sensation. The other period at which a distortion of sensory experience may occur, comes on during the phase of nerve regeneration when fibers are growing back into the area, but have not yet completely established their former connections. Both of these are illustrated in Henry Head's classical experiment on his own sensory nerves.

On April 25, 1903, two cutaneous nerves (ramus superficialis nervi radialis and nervi cutaneous antibrachii lateralis) of Head's left forearm were surgically divided near the elbow. The cut ends were immediately drawn together with silk sutures. On the following morning the radial half of the back of the hand and dorsal surface of the thumb were found to be insensitive to stimulation with cotton wool, to pricking with a pin, and to all degrees of heat and cold. The area insensitive to cotton wool extended slightly farther toward the ulnar aspect of the hand than that of the cutaneous analgesia. Between the two lay a narrow zone, where a painful stimulus produced a more unpleasant sensation than over the normal skin. The deeper structures of the forearm and hand were sensitive to pressures which deformed the overlying skin and the point of contact could be localized quite accurately. An excess of pressure produced an aching pain. Other than this deep sensibility, the area of distribution of the two superficial nerves was anesthetic. By the forty-third day after the operation it was noted that although there was no appreciable alteration of the area insensitive to cotton wool, the area of cutaneous analgesia was less extensive. As time went on the area of analgesia became progressively smaller, and by the eighty-sixth day the back of the hand was superficially sensitive to stimuli of moderate intensity, although the boundaries of the region insensitive to cotton wool stimulation remained relatively unaltered. From this time on, for a period of several months, the back of his hand was sensitive to pain, cold, heat and contact which moved the hairs, but the quality of the sensations elicited was peculiarly unpleasant, and quite unlike any sensation Head had previously experienced.

This phase of returning sensation during nerve regeneration was termed by Head, "protopathic sensibility." During this phase it was apparent that the threshold of stimulation was higher than that of normal skin, but when a sensation was elicited it was unpleasant, diffuse and difficult to localize. The "sensation of a point" which normally is felt when a sharp instrument is pressed on skin (not hard enough to produce pain) was not appreciated in the protopathic area. Only when pressure was sufficient to evoke pain was the contact felt at all, and then Head was conscious of a diffuse pain, which might be ascribed to an area at some distance from the actual point of contact. Light touch sensations came back fairly soon in hairy areas, but was promptly lost when the part had been shaved.

No return of sensation to any form of thermal stimulus could be discovered until one hundred twelve days after the operation. Thereafter cold spots and heat spots appeared in a somewhat irregular fashion, but it was not until months later that the middle ranges of temperature could be appreciated. Only when sensibility to light touch, the ability to recognize two compass points simultaneously applied, and to appreciate the middle ranges of temperature, had become well established did the unpleasant features of the protopathic phase disappear, and the ability to localize a stimulus become exact.

The finer grades of sensibility which accompany the final phase of nerve regeneration were termed by Head, "epicritic." Epicritic sensibility comprises the appreciation and localization of light touch, independent of hair; the recognition of two-dimensional stimulation; and the appreciation of temperatures between 27° and 38° C. These qualities of cutaneous sensibility, which depend upon the individual's ability to discriminate and localize accurately, are always the last to return after a nerve regenerates. Even after they seem well established, cooling of the part may abolish them, and then sensation promptly reverts to the protopathic type. Not only are the epicritic sensibilities last to return, but they are the qualities that are most prone to remain permanently deficient after a nerve regenerates. In Head's case the return of these qualities was unusually good, but even so, a small area on the dorsum of his hand in the region of the interosseous space between the index and middle finger metacarpals, failed to establish normal epicritic sensibility, and five years after the operation this area was still responding to stimuli with sensations that were characteristically protopathic.

From these, and supplementary observations Henry Head came to the conclusion that superficial sensibility was made up of two parts which he decided must be subserved by two distinct types of nerve fiber. The kind of fiber underlying protopathic sensibility he judged was a fast-growing, more primitive type that subserved the cruder aspects of sensation; while the fibers supplying epicritic sensibility were phylogenetically of more recent acquisition. He believed that epicritic sensibility normally exerted an inhibitory influence over the more primitive protopathic sensibility; and that only when this inhibitory influence was not present did the characteristic protopathic sensibility become apparent.

One of the most interesting observations which Head made in regard to protopathic sensibility was that it had many characteristics in common with visceral sensibility. In his earliest paper, written in conjunction with Rivers and Sherren [47] in 1905, the term "protopathic" was introduced and the suggestion was made that the nerves responsible for the sensory disturbances might be afferent units of the sympathetic nervous system. These authors said: "Now, one of the peculiarities of protopathic sensibility is the rapid restoration of the mechanism upon which it is based. This it shares with the sympathetic system. Moreover, when a peripheral nerve to the hand is divided, it is noticeable that the palm begins to sweat at a time after union which coincides approximately with that of the return of protopathic sensibility. This sweating is due to the motor fibres of the sympathetic (the 'autonomic fibres' of Langley) that supply the skin. It will therefore be no adventurous guess to suppose that the system we have called protopathic in the skin is one with the afferent fibres of the sympathetic as they supply the viscera. In both cases the sensation is badly localized, radiates widely, and is frequently referred to parts other than those stimulated. Both systems are incapable of appreciating light touch, and both are insensitive to the minor degrees of heat and cold. Both regenerate with the same rapidity and completeness. We wish, therefore, to put forward

a new conception of the nature of the afferent fibres in peripheral nerves. The whole body within and without is supplied
by the protopathic system. The fibres of this system in the skin
may be spoken of as somatic, those to the internal organs as
visceral protopathic fibres. Thus we shall no longer speak of
the afferent sympathetic system, but of the protopathic supply
of internal organs."

I have been unable to find a reference to this interpretation
in Head's writings subsequent to 1905, and it is possible that
he abandoned the idea that protopathic and sympathetic nerves
were identical in type. Whether or not he changed his mind
is immaterial for the moment. The importance of the quotation for my present purpose, is that it indicates how much
impressed Head was by the similarity between protopathic and
visceral sensibility. Many other investigators have been struck
by this similarity. It has been further pointed out that both
of these have a remarkable resemblance to the sensations
aroused by stimulation of the deeper somatic tissues, and to
those elicited from cases suffering from the "thalamic syndrome." There is something very suggestive about this resemblance of sensory experiences set up by four quite different
lesions. Lewis [68] has been impressed by this resemblance, and
in his text he has suggested that pain from deep somatic tissues,
the internal viscera, and that elicited from areas lacking in
touch sensibility, may be identical. In discussing Head's protopathic sensibility he says: "I suggest that the pain nerves are
derived from the deep, and not from the superficial system
and that to this the disagreeable and diffuse nature of the pain
are due," and again, in speaking of visceral pain: "To summa-
rise broadly, there is a general afferent supply common to
deep-lying somatic and to certain visceral structures; pain arising from one or the other is derived from the direct stimulation

of a common system of pain nerves, namely, the nerves of deep pain described in Chapter III. The pain impulses are identical with, or are generally associated with, afferent impulses that set up reflexly a common series of motor and sensory reactions. It is largely a matter of indifference whether the nerve fibres stimulated supply visceral or deep-lying somatic tissues; it is a matter of indifference whether they pass to the posterior roots by way of an anatomical path grouped as somatic or sympathetic; the result will depend (apart from strength and duration of stimulus) chiefly upon the segmental derivation of the afferent fibres concerned."

The resemblance between deep somatic pain, visceral pain and protopathic pain is thought-provoking. The further observation that these three types of peripheral pain possess qualities that are similar to those occurring in the thalamic syndrome, is even more remarkable because this latter type is of central origin. In all of these conditions there may be noted a dissociation between touch and pain, and a characteristic over-reaction to stimulation. The threshold to stimulation may be raised, but there is an explosive and peculiarly unpleasant reaction to relatively innocuous stimuli. Localization may be deficient and there is a tendency for the sensation to be referred to other areas than the point stimulated. All of the discriminative sensibilities may be impaired. These qualities may not all be present simultaneously or to the same degree during the regeneration of nerves or in the thalamic syndrome. Nor is it possible to state that the apparent resemblances between the several types of pain are significant of any fundamental relationship in their underlying mechanisms. But if there is such a relationship between central pain and those of peripheral origin, it is unnecessary to invent any new type of peripheral nerve to account for them.

Head's original experiment has been repeated many times by many different individuals who were impressed by the desirability of having a trained observer record his own sensory experiences. The principal findings reported by Head have been confirmed, although in their desire to refute Head's notion of a special, primitive type of nerve to account for protopathic pain, many observers have tended to emphasize the differences in their findings rather than the similarities. Heringa and Boeke [50] made a histologic study of segments of skin removed during the protopathic phase of returning sensibility, and found that the end-organs were beginning to regenerate throughout the skin. They ascribed the protopathic sensibility to the stimulation of these partially restored end-organs. Sharpey-Schäfer [105] felt that the abnormal sensations were "referred" peripherally from the site of nerve section, exactly as painful sensations may be referred into a phantom limb from the cut nerves of the stump. Stopford [114] confirmed Head's finding of a two-stage recovery of superficial sensibility, and added the fact that deep sensibility also exhibits a similar two-stage recovery. He explained the phenomena by pointing out that the distortion of the intraneural pattern, which must inevitably take place after a complete division and resuture of a cut nerve, results in fibers growing down neurilemmal paths to entirely different endings from those with which they were previously connected. The messages reaching the higher centers would thus be garbled. Stopford felt that the impulses reaching the higher centers might be capable of registering the cruder aspects of sensation in the thalamus, but that a complete re-education of the individual would be necessary before the finer discriminative judgments could be made concerning the sensory impressions coming from the involved part.

Trotter and Davies [119] carried out a careful study of sensory experiences following the surgical interruption of their own nerves. In one or the other of these men, seven different sensory nerves were divided, a small segment of the trunk was removed and the ends immediately resutured. Their studies gained in value, not only because of the number of nerves studied, but from the fact that these two trained observers were able to compare their subjective experiences throughout the experiment. When they used the same methods for testing skin sensibility that Head employed, their findings were essentially similar to his, but by using additional testing methods they were able to demonstrate factual differences that threw doubt on Head's interpretations, in particular, on his postulation of special protopathic nerves. The principal features of their findings that differed from those reported by Head, have been well summarized by Walshe.[120] Trotter and Davies were of the opinion that the most important alteration in sensibility of the skin after nerve section was due to a "hyperalgesia of recovery," which tended to modify what would otherwise be a simple diminution in sensory acuity resulting from a reduction in the numbers of functioning end-organs in the affected area of skin. In their experiments it was noted that the hyperalgesia was not constantly present, that it was observed at three different times after nerve section, and might represent different kinds of hyperalgesia, due to different causes. Immediately following the nerve section, the borders of the affected area were unduly sensitive for the first one or two days, and then this hyperesthesia disappeared. About a week later, rather suddenly, the intermediate zone again became hyperesthetic. There was a tendency for the sensitiveness to spread proximally along the superficial veins. This second hyperesthesia persisted for several weeks, but usually disappeared a short time before the third type appeared synchronously with the evidence that the sensory nerves were extending into the formerly anesthetic zone. This final stage of hyperesthesia corresponded in time to the protopathic phase of regeneration noted by Head. The first stage of hyperesthesia they felt might be due to several possible sources—the irritating effect of the nerve suture, the local inflammatory reaction set up by the operation, and possibly some minor degrees of phlebitis involving the superficial veins. The later stages of hyperesthesia they attributed to some irritative influence from the nerve itself. They considered the possibility that had been suggested by von Frey,[34] i.e., that some central activity set up by influences from the nerve lesion might be responsible for the altered sensibility of the area, but rejected it in favor of the view that the condition was due to peripheral changes in the tissues, taking place distal to the point of nerve section.

Although Trotter and Davies concluded that touch was little affected during nerve regeneration except as would be consistent with a loss of many end-organs subserving this sensation, they showed that cold, pain and the pain element of heat were intensified during nerve regeneration, and that sensations elicited from the involved area were referred to points at a distance from the point of stimulation. In explanation of these observations they say: "The evidence therefore seems to be tending in the direction of the view that both the qualitative peculiarities of sensation during recovery and the phenomenon of reference, the two great characteristics of sensibility in a recovering area, are related to some special feature in the circumstances of the regenerating nerve fibres which renders these latter abnormally accessible to stimuli."

The controversies that have developed as a result of differences in the interpretation of the factual data derived from clinical experiments on regenerating nerves, have all been

stimulating to the progress of understanding of pain mechanisms. It is not feasible to undertake a further discussion of
individual differences of opinion, nor is it possible to give a
final answer to the problem of protopathic pain, but it seems
worth while to call attention to some of the factual observations drawn from these experiments that must be taken into
account in making any interpretation.

1. There is a remarkable difference to be observed in the
behavior of sensory nerves that have been *physiologically* interrupted, in contrast to those that have been *surgically* sectioned.
When a nerve has been completely divided, no matter how
carefully the severed ends are brought together, there always
is a long delay in the recovery of sensibility in the anesthetic
part; complete recovery of normal sensibility is never assured;
and during the process of regeneration, a distortion of sensibility of some degree (protopathic phase) is invariably present.
In contrast with this, a more physiologic interruption of a
nerve, as by crushing with a forceps, that does not disrupt its
internal relationships or completely sever the nerve sheath,
though it produces the same area of temporary anesthesia, has
quite different results. The period of delay in recovery of
sensation is much shorter; the protopathic phase of distorted
sensibility is lacking; and a complete restoration of normal
sensation is almost certain to follow. This observation, emphasized by Stopford,[114] indicates that a distortion of intraneural
pattern of fiber arrangement probably has something to do
with the protopathic phase and with the ability of a sensory
nerve to rapidly and completely establish its former functions.

2. When, after section of a sensory nerve, normal (epicritic)
sensory perception begins to be established, cooling of the
part causes it to revert to the phase of protopathic sensibility.
This observation indicates that changes in the physiologic status

of the nerve fibers and their endings may result in distortions of sensory patterns as they are registered at the perceptual level. There is good physiologic evidence to support the view that sensory dissociation can occur by changing the physiologic state of a normal sensory nerve trunk. An outstanding example of this is seen during the phase of complete loss of touch sense when a segment of nerve is asphyxiated by depriving it of its blood supply for a time with a sphygmomanometer cuff. With the loss of this part of the pattern of sensory impulses, a distortion of sensory perception, similar to that of protopathic sensibility, may be demonstrated.

3. In Head's experiment there were two areas of skin which were of special interest. One of these was found on the wrist soon after the nerve section had been accomplished. In this small triangle the skin was insensitive to prick and other forms of painful stimuli but remained sensitive to stimulation with cotton wool. The existence of such an area, exhibiting an exactly opposite response to stimulation to that observed elsewhere at the margins of the anesthetic area, was fortuitous, in that it probably represented an individual variation in the distribution of the nerve supply to that part. Its importance lies in the demonstration that individual variations exist which may act to confuse the findings in any particular experiment, and perhaps lead to erroneous conclusions. The second area of interest was an irregular triangle of skin on the dorsum of the hand over the index and middle finger metacarpals. This particular region did not regain normal sensibility, and five years after the nerve had been sectioned, it was still responding to stimulation with sensations typical of the protopathic phase of nerve regeneration. The persistence of this zone constitutes an argument against some of the interpretations that have been offered to explain the disturbance in sensory perception

during regeneration. For instance, if, as Sharpey-Schäfer contended, the distortions were due to irritation at the site of nerve section and referred peripherally, it is peculiar that such a reference remained confined to one small area so far removed from the point of nerve section. It is apparent, too, that this area of disturbance could not be due to nerve endings in the process of regeneration,[50] nor to contact of growing nerve fibers with non-neural tissue.[119] Furthermore, it is difficult to explain the persistence of this single area, if, as Stopford has contended, the establishment of normal sensibility is merely a question of re-education of the individual.

4. Perhaps the most interesting feature of Head's experiment was observable immediately after the nerve section. On the morning after the operation on his arm, Head observed that between the analgesic area and the normally innervated skin, lay a "narrow zone, where a painful stimulus produced a more unpleasant sensation than over normal skin." This observation has been repeatedly confirmed. The area of anesthesia that develops after the division of a nerve does not represent the full limits of sensory distribution of that nerve. The totally anesthetic zone is considerably smaller than would have been anticipated. Around it is an "intermediate zone" which responds to strong stimulation and the extremes of temperature, with painful sensation. Sometimes the fact that sensation can thus be elicited from areas within the anatomic boundaries of a nerve distribution has led surgeons to doubt that a nerve has been completely divided. But this finding is to be expected. It is due to the *overlap* in the distribution of sensory elements from other nerves supplying adjacent skin areas.

It is most difficult to account for the distortion of sensation in the overlap zone. It is conceivable that some change in the local tissue nutrition, or the liberation of "some irritating substance produced as the result of the division and degeneration of the nerve" (postulated by Trotter and Davies [119]), may modify the responses of the remaining end-organs in this area. It is also conceivable that the nerve fibers that overlap by the widest margins might represent a different type of neuron than those which supply the normally innervated skin. We might assume, as Head did in his original explanation of proto-pathic pain, that sympathetic afferents are supplied to the skin. It could further be assumed that these sympathetic fibers ar-borize more widely than do somatic afferents, and that they carry quite different messages. But in the absence of evidence supporting such an assumption, it seems more likely that a simple withdrawal of a part of the sensory receptors which register normal sensation, is the only change that has taken place locally. There is the possibility, to be discussed in the next chapter, that some chemical change may take place in the tissues secondary to the nerve section, but the only anatomic alteration at the periphery has been a loss of interdigitating sensory endings. It is possible, therefore, that any factor which tended to disturb the normal relationship between the various impulses subserving sensation might result in perceptual mis-interpretations.

This is an important assumption. If it can be justified, it furnishes a reasonable explanation for the altered sensibility of the overlap area, and a possible clue to an understanding of protopathic pain. The only feature that is common to both conditions is that of "incompleteness," i.e., in each case, the stimulation of the involved area fails to initiate the full com-posite of impulses that are customarily aroused by that same stimulus under "normal" conditions. Weddell [123] apparently believes that such a possibility is consistent with his anatomic findings, because he says: "In the course of regeneration, nerve fibres will arrive at each separate spot at different times, because they approach it from different directions and the ultimate course to be followed by the individual fibres will necessarily be of different lengths. Thus, in the course of regeneration there will be a phase in which each sensory spot is innervated by a single fibre instead of multiple fibres. During this phase there will be no anatomical basis for spatial summation; therefore reactions to stimuli will tend to conform to an 'all or nothing' law, leading to the characteristic explosive type of sensation, and there can be no recognition of gradation and no possibility of accurate localization"—and: "The same thing is seen in so-called 'intermediate zones,' those areas of diminished sensibility which are found in the zones of overlap between peripheral sensory nerves after section or anaesthetization. In these areas there is an alteration in sensibility which tends to have an irradiating quality, localization is extremely poor, and so is two-point discrimination and the recognition of figure patterns traced on the skin. Moreover, histological observations have shown the presence of isolated Meissner's corpuscles and subcutaneous nerve nets in skin from a patient with a partial interruption of the ulnar nerve who displayed an alteration in sensibility similar to that just described."

Since sensory perception is dependent upon the pattern of central excitation registered by the impulses coming from the periphery, it follows that anything that might act to disturb the normal pattern of impulses anywhere along their route from the periphery to the perceptual centers might lead to an unusual pattern of central excitation, and hence produce abnormal changes in sensory experience. In other words, if we are justified in assuming that a simple withdrawal of a part of the peripheral end-organs can alter sensation, there should be other factors between the periphery and the sensorium that might produce similar alterations. Theoretically then, one might expect to observe sensory disturbances of some degree in any or all of the following conditions: partial loss of local sensibility; a partial injury to a sensory nerve; during nerve regeneration; in an overlap area; as a result of any distortion of intraneural pattern; a blockade to part of the conducting fibers in the posterior root; a pathological state of the inter-nuncial pool within the spinal cord; and any lesion within the central nervous system that affected parts of the pathways conducting sensory impulses, without equally involving them all. Clinical experience would indicate that all of the peripheral conditions enumerated *may* distort sensation, and the distortions are unpleasant if not actually painful. And in the course of the following discussion of hyperalgesia, it will be noted that certain lesions within the spinal cord are even more prone to disturb normal sensibility.

CHAPTER XIII

*Hyperalgesia*

Any injury that directly or indirectly involves the sensory nerves may lead to the development of an abnormal sensitiveness of the skin. All sensory experiences derived from the skin may be altered in this condition, so that it is frequently called a "hyperesthesia," or a "hyperpathia." However, since the principal alteration in sensibility is an intensification of pain sensation it is more commonly referred to as a "hyperalgesia." In this state the tissues are unduly sensitive and they tend to react to the most innocuous stimuli with explosive sensations of pain accompanied by withdrawal reflexes. When the hyperalgesia is extreme in the causalgic states, even blowing one's breath across the skin surface causes vivid sensations of pain and an uncontrollable impulse to jerk away from the stimulus.

The mechanism underlying hyperalgesia is obscure, and the problems pertaining to it are intimately related to many of the other problems that have been previously considered. The difficulty encountered in adequately presenting the problem of hyperalgesia is complicated by the fact that it can be induced by a number of quite different lesions. The irritation of a foreign body, the crushing of a bit of skin, the irritation of a sensory nerve, strychninization of the posterior horn of gray matter of the cord, lesions involving the posterior columns, injuries to the cervical portion of the spinal cord, and suprathalamic lesions, can all bring about a peripheral hyperalgesia. It is possible that the hyperalgesic states resulting from these different lesions may not all be of the same type, but the similarity in clinical manifestations seen in each, suggests that they all have a common denominator. At the present time there is no unanimity of opinion as to what this underlying factor may be.

The easiest way to produce a local hyperalgesia experimentally is to pick up a small piece of skin in a tooth forceps and give it a single strong pinch. Within a few minutes of the time of injury there develops around this area, and sometimes extending for a considerable distance distal to the site of the original pinch, a typical, superficial hyperalgesia. The change in pain sensibility which characterizes this condition may persist for hours or days. Gellhorn [42] has shown that, in addition to the exaggeration of the disagreeable quality of sensations elicited by stimulation, there is an accompanying disturbance of the ability to localize the point of stimulation. Stimuli which are very accurately localized over normally innervated skin, are either inaccurately localized when applied to the hyperalgesic area or are ascribed to areas at an appreciable distance away from the point of stimulation. Gellhorn believes that the spinal cord centers are implicated in the altered condition of the skin, and refers to the phenomena as "spinal irradiation." Echlin and Propper [23] have shown that a preliminary scraping of a frog's skin caused an increase in the frequency of nerve impulses conducted along sensory fibers as the result of simple pressure stimuli. Their work implies that injuries of the skin "hypersensitize" it, that is, produce some alteration in the skin itself, so that an afferent impulse set up by relatively innocuous contacts are altered in character. Lewis [69] has conducted an extensive and important series of experiments relating to hyperalgesia. His studies indicate that as a result of injury, the tissues elaborate a certain unknown

substance which acts to render the sensory nerve-endings
hyperexcitable. He has shown that when the skin is involved in
the hyperalgesic state, the response to warmth is enhanced, and
the sensation experienced by the subject is similar to that

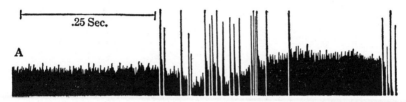

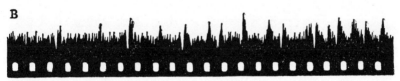

FIG. 23.—DORSAL CUTANEOUS NERVE OF THE FROG

*A*, Large rapid potential waves due to touch; *B*, After the surface layers of the
skin had been removed by scraping, a crush gives discharge consisting entirely of
slow impulses.

*Note.* The rate at which the individual potential wave is completed is a measure
of the rate at which it is traveling past the electrodes. (From Adrian: *Proc. Roy.
Soc.* London, s, B. 1931, 109; 1.)

aroused by subjecting his normal skin to much higher temperatures. The sensations elicited from the hyperalgesic area
by pricking, light friction and any change that increases local
tension, are more intense, and protective reflexes may be exaggerated.

The extent of skin involvement in the hyperalgesic state resulting from local injury seems to vary according to the degree
of injury, but the process, according to Lewis, remains within
the distribution of a single peripheral nerve or one of its
branches, and never extends into the territory of adjacent
nerves. If the skin is first infiltrated with novocaine, the ex-

perimental crushing injury is painless, and the development
of the hyperalgesia is delayed until the anesthetic effect has
worn off. If, instead of a direct injury to the skin, a sensory
nerve branch is stimulated, exactly the same type of spreading
hyperalgesia develops. When the nerve has been blocked with
novocaine above the site of its stimulation the hyperalgesia
does not appear until after the blockade has disappeared.
When the branch is blocked by the local anesthetic at a point
distal to the point of stimulation, hyperalgesia develops around
the site of stimulation but does not spread beyond the
blockade area, even after the anesthetic effect of the novocaine
has gone.

These observations demonstrate that nerve impulses play an
essential role in the development of the hyperalgesic state. Since
Lewis was able to produce this state in human subjects de-
prived of a normal sympathetic nerve supply, he has concluded
that the sympathetic nerves are not essential to the process;
nor does he think that motor neurons of the anterior horn play
any part in it. The phenomenon can be elicited as long as the
neurons of the posterior root remain intact.

Lewis has come to the conclusion that hyperalgesia is mediated by hitherto unrecognized neurons in the posterior root
ganglia, which he has called "nocifensors." He believes that
they are distinct from the sensory nerves because they are
affected by asphyxia and cocaine differently than are the
sensory nerves. Thus cocaine paralyzes the pain fibers before
it interferes with the development of hyperalgesia; while asphyxia has an opposite effect, paralyzing the fibers responsible
for hyperalgesia before it has an appreciable effect on pain conduction. He further points out that the widespread influence
exerted by the nocifensors implies that there is a wide arboriza-
tion of individual fibers, and he argues that if the ordinary

sensory fibers arborized to this extent, accurate localization would be impossible. He visualizes a single nocifensor neuron as having its cell body in a posterior root ganglion, and its branching fibers extending widely in the distribution of one

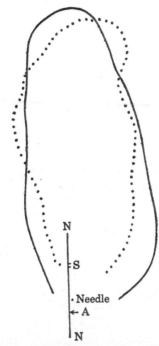

FIG. 24.—STIMULATION OF NERVE THROUGH SKIN, NERVE BLOCKED ABOVE

The course of the anterior branch of the external cutaneous nerve had been marked on the left forearm days before.

0 min.   The region of the nerve injected (at *A*) with 1 cc. 1 per cent novocaine, the needle being inserted where shown.

5 min.   The resultant area of anesthesia and hypesthesia has fully developed and is mapped out (dotted line).

9½ min.  Faradic stimulation at *S* in line of nerve for 2 min. Current of usual strength; goose skin throughout stimulation in surrounding skin. The current felt as a slight local tingle; no fluttering along the nerve. At the end of stimulation the area of anesthesia and hypesthesia is unchanged in extent and degree.

25 min.  The anesthesia and hypesthesia have disappeared and a large area of hyperalgesia has appeared (solid line). (From Lewis: Clin. Sc. 1936, 2, 387.)

particular peripheral nerve. He believes that these neuron units are closely identified with skin structure and that they are concerned with protective mechanisms rather than with localizable sensation. An injury to the skin or to a sensory nerve

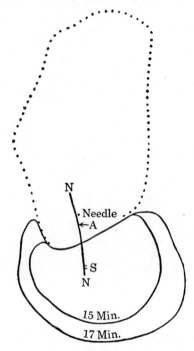

FIG. 25.—STIMULATION OF AN ANTERIOR BRANCH OF THE EXTERNAL CUTANEOUS
         NERVE (N) THROUGH SKIN; NERVE BLOCKED BELOW

0 min.    The region of the nerve was injected at *A* with 1 cc. of 1 per cent novocaine.

6 min.    Area of anesthesia and hypesthesia fully developed and mapped out (dotted line).

8 min.    Faradic stimulation at *S*, with coil at usual strength, for 2 min.; goose skin maintained in surrounding skin throughout. The stimulus very painful locally, and fluttering pain felt during the whole period along the nerve's territory.

15 min.   An area of hyperalgesia has developed around the point of stimulation and is charted.

17 min.   The nerve block is recovering. The area of hyperalgesia has increased a little.

19 min.   A little spontaneous burning felt around region of stimulation, but nowhere else; the nerve block has quite recovered and skin sensation in the corresponding area is perfectly normal and remains so for the next hour of observation. (From Lewis: Clin. Sc. 1936, 2, 386.)

is supposed to activate the nocifensors to bring about changes in the skin, leading to the elaboration of a relatively stable metabolite which acts to lower the threshold for stimulation of pain-conducting sensory neurons.

Lewis's experimental studies are of great value in demonstrating two important points relating to hyperalgesic states. The first one is that the development of hyperalgesia is due, in part at least, to the elaboration of some substance within the skin itself, which alters its sensibility. The second one is that this change in the skin is mediated by nerve impulses. His observations may throw some light on the observations of Mitchell [85] and Tinel [116] to the effect that, in some cases, pain has been relieved by cutting a nerve *distal* to the lesion of the nerve trunk that is apparently causing the pain. I have never cut a nerve distal to the lesion to test this observation, but I have injected novocaine solution distal to a nerve lesion in a case suffering from causalgia and secured a temporary alleviation of symptoms. It is also possible that these peripheral effects produced by nerve irritation may have some relation to the trophic changes in tissue structure that have been such a puzzling feature of many pain syndromes.

No one has seriously challenged Lewis's observations, but doubts have been expressed as to the necessity for his postulation of special nerves to account for them. Walshe [120] has made a critical review of the literature dealing with the anatomy and physiology of cutaneous sensibility. In it he has objected to the "nocifensor" concept, and with even more force to Head's "protopathic" nerves. He has subjected the theories of both Lewis and Head to a minute dissection and concludes that in neither case are the theories necessitated by the factual observations that have been reported. Walshe finds it difficult to construct a diagram of a nocifensor unit on the basis of Lewis's writings since its functions are presumably accomplished by its terminal plexus whose endings act as both receptors and effectors. He says: "No discoverable function can be conceived for a central prolongation of the nocifensor system into the central nervous system, for of itself the system subserves no sensory function, and its activities are locally engendered and locally executed in the skin."

I must confess to a similar difficulty in understanding the anatomy of the nocifensor unit if its impulses spread through the peripheral nerve net without involving the nerve cell or its spinal connections. For instance, let us start with the assumption that an injury involving a nocifensor unit of the radial nerve may cause a hyperalgesia spreading throughout the territory of this nerve, but not extending into the territory of either the ulnar or the median nerves. The radial nerve is related to several posterior roots. If one is constructing a diagram of the nocifensor unit involved by the injury, in which of these different posterior root ganglia is the cell body of the unit to be placed? If each posterior root ganglion related to the radial nerve contains one or more nocifensor nerve cells, how is the impulse from the unit originally activated, going to spread to involve them all? Do they form peripheral anastomoses, one with the other throughout the distribution of each nerve, or do they overlap so extensively that a single local lesion in any part of the radial distribution will activate terminals of each one of them simultaneously? And if they branch or intercommunicate to this extent, how does it happen that the hyperalgesia remains so strictly confined to the radial nerve distribution, as Lewis states that it does?

These are academic questions, yet they illustrate some of the difficulties encountered in forming an accurate visualization of a nocifensor unit. They seem to indicate, too, that the central extensions of whatever nerve unit is activated in the production of hyperalgesia, *do* function, and that it is by way of central connections that the process spreads to involve wider and wider areas. And once it is conceded that the activities of nocifensor units involve their central connections, the necessity for their postulation is gone, because exactly the same functions might be served by sensory nerves already known to exist. In fact, the anatomic characteristics of the subepithelial nerve net which has been described by Woollard [129] and Weddell [123] as subserving pain sensation, would fulfill all the requirements demanded by Lewis to explain the activities he has ascribed to the nocifensors. In addition, the neurophysiologist has demonstrated that centripetal impulses traversing sensory nerves may represent true reflexes, completed within the spinal cord, instead of "axon reflexes." *

* Tönnies has recently shown that following the stimulation of a sensory nerve, such as the internal saphenous, there occurs a centrifugal discharge of impulses back down this same nerve. He has demonstrated that a considerable percentage of the total number of sensory fibers of the nerve (including some of the fastest conducting fibers) are involved in this discharge. He was able to prove that this activity did not represent an axon reflex, but was the result of true reflexes taking place within the spinal cord. He found that when one saphenous nerve was stimulated, the "posterior root reflexes," as recorded from that same nerve, exhibited all the phenomena of summation, inhibition, etc., which characterize true reflexes, and he was able to record similar, but somewhat diminished discharges passing centrifugally along the opposite saphenous nerve or adjacent posterior roots. When simultaneous records were taken from both internal saphenous nerves after the stimulation of one of them, the nature of the reflex discharge over each nerve was identical with the other, and impulses in the nerve contralateral to the point of stimulation were delayed by an interval that corresponded to the time required for the impulses to pass over one or two additional synapses within the spinal cord.

At the present time, of course, it is impossible to say whether or not posterior root reflexes have any relation to hyperalgesia, or any other clinical state. Anderson, Dow and Livingston [3] attempted to show that a chronic irritative lesion of one hind leg of a dog brought about changes in the posterior root reflexes in the saphenous nerve of that side, but failed. However, Tönnies' demonstration of centrifugal impulses in large numbers passing out from the spinal cord by way of the posterior roots and sensory nerves is of great interest, and the fact that such discharges may involve adjacent or contralateral sensory nerves suggests that this mechanism, or one of a similar nature may eventually prove to be the basis for explaining the spread of clinical signs and symptoms from the original site of injury to involve neighboring nerves or those of the contralateral extremity. ("Mirror image.")

There are other reasons for questioning the nocifensor concept in its exclusion of a central participation in the production of hyperalgesia. In the causalgic states, as I have observed them, the hyperalgesia is rarely confined to the distribution of a single nerve, and in some cases the whole extremity is involved in the process even though the lesion initiating it is represented by a minor injury of but one nerve. Such a spread is difficult to account for on the basis of strictly peripheral units confined to the distribution of single nerves. Furthermore, it is well known that lesions within the central nervous system can bring about a cutaneous hyperalgesia which is very similar to, if not identical with, that caused by peripheral nerve irritation.

Dusser de Barenne [21] has shown that hyperalgesia can be induced by injecting small amounts of strychnine into the posterior horns of gray matter of the spinal cord. The strychnine apparently acts directly on the cell bodies of neurons rather than upon nerve fibers. Therefore, even though nocifensors might be conceived of as sending dendritic processes into the posterior horns, it is hardly likely that the strychnine affects them directly. Apparently the sensitization of neurons within the spinal cord is able to bring about some secondary peripheral effect, or acts to alter the shunting of incoming sensory impulses. This latter explanation seems to be the more probable one, since injuries to other parts of the spinal cord or brain may, in certain instances, produce a peripheral hyperalgesia.

A good example of this is seen in clinical cases of the "thalamic syndrome" in which large areas of the body surface may develop hyperalgesia. Head and Holmes [48] have assumed that the essential lesion in this thalamic syndrome was an interruption of the corticothalamic projections, and that thereby the inhibitory influence exerted by the cortex over thalamic responses was removed. The evidence in support of the view that the thalamus is the center for "affective states" and is normally under the control of an inhibitory influence from the cortex has been repeatedly questioned. Lashley [62] has reviewed the evidence supporting this view and concludes that such an interpretation of clinical observations is not justified. Mahoney [79] removed a part of the sensory cortex of a patient suffering from phantom limb pain. According to Head's view such a procedure would remove cortical inhibition and might be expected to increase the pain. Instead the pain was relieved. And the fact that hyperalgesic states similar to those observed in the thalamic syndrome, may occur as a result of central lesions occurring at lower levels, is further evidence against this interpretation.

Lesions of the posterior columns may produce hyperalgesia at the periphery. There has been a good deal of discussion as to why this should be so. The most reasonable assumption seems to be that the sensory impulses conducted by the posterior columns tend to modify those conducted by the spinothalamic tract. Under normal circumstances, the impulses conducted by these two sensory pathways reach the sensorium to establish a pattern of excitation that results in "normal" sensation. But when the impulses subserving touch and pressure are interrupted, a distortion of sensation results in which only the cruder and more unpleasant aspects of sensory experience are present.*

* This concept has been emphasized by Riddoch.[101] The following quotation is taken from his excellent discussion of "central pain."

"Under normal conditions, one method by which pain is kept in abeyance appears to be through the activity of the neural mechanism concerned with those aspects of sensation which are called discriminative and it is adequate so long as the pain receptors are not massively stimulated. . . . Even before they reach the optic thalamus and cerebral cortex to disturb consciousness, all sensory impulses undergo repeated

Zotterman [130] has added some observations, based on a study of spike heights of axone potentials taken from the saphenous nerve of the cat, which have influenced him to believe that a central inhibitory effect is exerted on "protopathic" fibers by "epicritic" fibers within the spinal cord. He subscribes to Foerster's view that the hyperalgesia resulting from lesions of the dorsal columns is due to "an exclusion of the highly differentiated and phylogenetically younger system of cutaneous sensory fibres, which normally exert an inhibitory influence upon the very ancient system of pain fibres." In speaking of tickle and itching, which he thinks are related to pain, he says: "Thus it seems that the fast impulses traveling up the posterior columns inhibit the central effect of the later arriving impulses. The less the large, fast fibers are stimulated the more intense become the tickling and itching sensations elicited by the slow impulses." Rubbing an itching or painful area is an instinctive reaction, and in many instances it seems to give some degree of relief. When one bumps his shin against a chair, the impulse to compress or rub the injured part is almost irresistible. Such a reaction is usually accompanied by tightening of the muscles, straining, biting the lips, or squeezing the hands together with painful force. Wolff, Hardy and Gooddell [126] have shown that this voluntary inducing of pain reaction from some other part of the body than that from which the original painful stimulus has arisen, has a definite effect on pain

---

modification, through the processes of integration. Under normal circumstances, the points are set, from the posterior horns upwards, in favour of all those impulses which arouse discriminative sensations—touch, pressure, posture, etc.; and it is only when stimulation of pain receptors is massive enough to overcome the inhibitory processes, that pain impulses become preponent. On the other hand, inhibition may be weakened by continued anxiety and general ill health and under these circumstances pain develops with abnormal ease.

"Pain of central origin, that is, from organic lesions of the sensory gray matter and tracts of the neuraxis, can be said to be the result of disintegration of the physiological processes which underlie sensory experience."

threshold. These authors have used thermal radiations to establish a pain threshold from the skin, and have shown that there is a remarkably constant threshold for different individuals, and for the same individual under most circumstances. However, "intense pain in any part of the body raised the threshold of the skin in other parts as much as 35%." Loud noises were shown to be capable of raising the pain threshold from 14 per cent to 32 per cent depending upon the duration of the stimulus, and the authors expressed the belief that other factors, "such as the excitement of a contest or accident would also exert appreciable effects on the reaction to pain."

All of these contributions tend to support the interpretation of pain as expressed in the opening chapters of the monograph. One of the essential features of this interpretation was that the impulses subserving pain are subject to modification anywhere between the periphery and the sensorium. It should now be possible to state with more assurance what some of these factors may be that contribute to the modification. One of these seems to be the elaboration in the skin of some chemical substance which acts to increase the sensitiveness of the skin locally. A second one may be represented by a simple withdrawal of a part of the impulses which customarily constitute the "composite" of impulses underlying "normal" sensations derived from the skin. A third one, apparently is dependent upon a distortion of intraneural pattern resulting from an anatomic interruption of nerve continuity, which results in fibers establishing new connections. It is quite possible that the disturbance of cutaneous sensibility observed in the "protopathic phase" of nerve regeneration may represent a combination of the first and third of these factors, while the altered sensibility of the "intermediate zone" may be a combination of the first two.

Added to these peripherally acting factors which tend to modify pain, are the equally important factors that act centrally. Among these might be mentioned an abnormal sensitivity of the cells of the posterior horn of gray matter, lesions of the posterior columns, or injuries to the brain in the region of the thalamus. And finally, anything that tends to alter the status of the internuncial pool in the receiving station at the cord level, or the integrated neuron systems of the perceptual centers in which the pattern of excitation registers, may act to modify pain sensations.

I am not assuming that these generalizations afford a final answer to any of the obscure problems that have been enumerated. But they point toward a working hypothesis which may be of assistance in interpreting clinical observations. My tendency is to emphasize, more and more, the importance of the central factors that modify pain, and I would use the concept of the "internuncial pool" to implement these factors.

## CHAPTER XIV

## *The Sympathetic Component*

Interest in the sympathetic nervous system and its functions has grown in recent years since it has been demonstrated that an increasingly large number of clinical conditions have been benefited by procedures that interrupt its pathways. Ganglion-ectomy has been used with considerable success in the treatment of thrombo-angiitis obliterans, Raynaud's disease, angina pectoris, Hirschsprung's disease, hypertension and a number of other clinical entities. Novocaine injection that produces a temporary interruption of sympathetic pathways, has been found useful as a prognostic test to determine the probable value of a subsequent sympathectomy, and more recently it has been employed as a therapeutic agent in its own right. It has proven to be of value in the treatment of deep venous thrombosis, and recent observations by Schumaker [108] suggest that it may be useful in controlling labor pain. A single novocaine blockade of the lumbar ganglia abolishes the pain due to uterine contractions for a period of four or five hours. In a series of sixteen cases, Schumaker has been able to control this element of the labor pains without materially reducing the strength of contraction of the uterus.

The general indications for an operation that interrupts the sympathetic pathway are based on two established facts—first, that these nerves regulate the tonus of blood vessels, and second, that sensory neurons conducting pain impulses from the internal organs, traverse the sympathetic chain to reach the spinal cord. The indications then would be—any condition in which there is reason to believe that a release of normal vaso-motor tonus, or of a definite vasospasm, would improve the local circulation sufficiently to counteract a threat to tissue nu-trition—and any pain from the internal organs which otherwise cannot be controlled. On the basis of this knowledge it is pos-sible to account for the beneficial results, and the relief from pain, that is conferred by a ganglionectomy, in many instances.

On the other hand, it is not always easy to account for the relief of symptoms in the causalgic states which involve pe-ripheral parts of the body and may not show any obvious threat to tissue nutrition. It is true that some surgeons ascribe the cure of symptoms, following a sympathectomy, to a cut-ting of pain pathways, which they believe traverse the gangli-onic chain to reach the spinal cord. Others ascribe the relief to some change in the vasomotor tonus of the peripheral blood vessels. Neither of these alternative explanations, however, is completely consistent with experimental and clinical data. In order to make this point clear it is necessary to consider briefly these alternatives in relation to the conflicting evidence from which they have been derived.

Leriche,[64] Foerster,[30] Reichert,[100] Fay,[25] and others are of the opinion that sensory fibers supplying the peripheral parts of the body may pass through the sympathetic ganglia to reach the cord. Slaughter [110] has reported a case that bears on this interpretation. In this case a transection of the spinal cord, con-firmed by a laminectomy, had occurred at the first lumbar seg-ment. The patient developed a severe burning and prickling pain ascribed to both lower extremities. The pain was relieved by a bilateral lumbar and sacral sympathetic ganglionectomy. This observation suggests that the pain impulses from the legs must have followed sympathetic pathways to reach the intact portion of the spinal cord above the first lumbar level.

However, the vast majority of experimental evidence fails to support this clinical interpretation. Carefully controlled laboratory experiments indicate that *all* pain impulses from the extremities are carried by fibers which go directly to the spinal cord by way of the posterior roots, without entering the sympathetic chain. For a long time I was inclined to doubt this dictum of the laboratory workers. I suspected that perhaps the reason no pain impulses appeared to pass through the sympathetic chain might be due to a failure to stimulate *visceral* afferent neurons. With this possibility in mind, Burget and I [10] attempted, in 1931, to show that impulses of painful intensity from the major blood vessels might follow sympathetic pathways. We divided the posterior roots of the brachial plexus of one forelimb in a number of dogs. This operation interrupted the usual pathways for pain conduction, but left a possible route to the cord by way of the gray rami and the sympathetic chain, whereby pain impulses might reach the central nervous system. Lactic acid in dilute solution was injected into the peripheral arteries of the de-afferenated limb. This fluid, injected into an artery of a control animal elicited evidence of severe pain, but no response in the animals whose posterior roots had been divided. Our observations were in line with previous experimental findings, and since then Moore and Singleton [88] have submitted more conclusive evidence to the same effect, i.e., that pain impulses from blood vessels as well as all other peripheral tissues, reach the spinal cord without passing through the sympathetic chain. Hinsey,[53] who is particularly well qualified to pass on this question, states: "There is no evidence, either clinical or experimental, which will stand critical analysis, to support the view that pain impulses from the extremities reach the spinal cord by way of the sympathetic ganglia." In view of all of these considerations, and unless better evidence is forthcoming, it is not reasonable to ascribe the benefit conferred by sympathectomy in the causalgic states to an interruption of pain pathways.

The second interpretation is more consistent with established facts relating to the sympathetic nerves. It is known that these nerves maintain a constant tonic influence on the peripheral blood vessels and are capable of causing a sustained vasospasm. It might be assumed, therefore, that the causalgic pain is produced by a local ischemia which a release from the sympathetic influence tends to counteract. In commenting on causalgia, Lewis [68] has said: "According to Leriche, the pain of causalgia may be abolished by sympathectomy. A case coming within my own observation convinces me that he is right; both pain and tenderness may disappear very quickly after this operation. The action is unclear. Sympathectomy leaves the sensation in the normal unaltered, a fact easy to determine in the skin of those sympathectomized. When skin pain and tenderness such as typify causalgia disappear after sympathectomy, it is hardly open to us to suppose that sensory nerve fibres passing from skin to spinal cord have been divided. Similarly, it is difficult to suppose that relief comes through interruption of nocifensor nerve paths—for normal nocifensor reactions in skin are likewise uninfluenced by sympathectomy—unless we accept the improbable idea that nocifensor fibres traverse the sympathetic chain on the way to the periphery and have their cell stations at a lower level. Thus a process of reasonable exclusion would seem to bring us to the view that when sympathectomy relieves causalgia it does so by depriving the skin of sympathetic nerve supply; persistently increased bloodflow through the cutaneous vessels consequent upon loss of vasomotor tone appears to be the only way of explaining the relief that is consistent with our remaining knowledge."

I should like to be able to subscribe wholeheartedly to this interpretation because it seems to be the only reasonable alternative if I reject the view that ganglionectomy interrupts a pain pathway. But it does not seem to conform to my clinical observations. Nor does Lewis seem to be satisfied with the explanation. He points out in the same discussion that the skin temperature in certain cases of causalgia is higher than normal. Skin temperature may not be an accurate gauge of the nutrition of skin cells, but the raised temperature does not suggest a local ischemia, or the sort of impaired nutrition that produces burning pain in a digit undergoing early gangrenous changes.

I am not ruling out a vasomotor release as a possible factor in the cure of causalgia. Many of the cases which I consider as belonging to the causalgic states, have a lower temperature in the affected part than in the contralateral limb. It is reasonable to suppose that an increased blood supply might favorably alter the physiologic status of the sensory nerve endings. In the first cases that I was able to relieve of pain by a ganglionectomy, I noted the improved circulation and was satisfied that this was the explanation for the pain relief. Later this conviction was shaken by the observation that in certain instances the pain syndrome persisted in spite of an augmented circulation. The two following case summaries illustrate this point.

CASE No. 21.—Mr. J. H., aged 36, was examined in August, 1933, because of pain in his right foot. In 1932 a rolling lump of dirt struck the dorsum of his right foot just below, and anterior to, the external malleolus. X-ray plates did not reveal a fracture, and the injury was treated as a minor bruise. Some three weeks later it was noted that the slight swelling had persisted and the pain was increasing. Still later the toes began to "pull up over the top of the foot" and his leg tended to jerk uncontrollably when the pain was severe. The area of injury became so hyperesthetic that the weight of bed-covers, a light touch, or even a quick gesture toward the foot precipitated a paroxysm of pain that radiated up the extremity to the hip. He could tolerate firm pressure better than light touch. The whole foot was hyperesthetic, but there was a brownish spot about the size of a dime just in front of the malleolus that was exquisitely sensitive. The foot was colder than normal, the skin thin and glistening, the joints stiff, the toes drawn up and the foot was atrophied. X-ray plates revealed an osteoporosis.

A lumbar ganglionectomy was attempted but exposure was inadequate and only one ganglion was removed. The operation was followed by a pulmonary atelectasis. For three weeks the foot remained warm and free from pain. Then the pain recurred. A few months later the head of the fifth metatarsal was removed without lessening his complaints. Then in succession the different nerves to the foot were surgically interrupted at the ankle level. The first important nerve to be divided was the posterior tibial. There followed an immediate and persistent warming of the foot. There was every evidence that the local tissue nutrition had improved. The pain was relieved for a week, and then, in spite of the continued warmth of the foot, it recurred with its original intensity. After each nerve was divided there would be a temporary lessening of the pain, and then it would return. Just why the division of all of the nerves of the foot did not relieve pain that seemed to come from an area distal to the point at which each one was divided, is not clear. Apparently the nerve section was not done at a distance high enough above the source of the pain, because an amputation of the leg three inches below the knee stopped the pain permanently and completely.

CASE No. 22.—Mr. J. S., a 20-year-old bus driver, was struck on the dorsum of the right wrist. There was no fracture and the injury was not considered serious. But his complaints increased and a year after the accident he was still unable to work. The wrist was reasonably comfortable only when bandaged firmly to a cock-up splint. The hand was dusky, cold, damp and hyperesthetic. His joints were stiff, the muscles weak, and the bones showed an advanced degree of osteoporosis. Local injections of novocaine into a particularly tender spot on the dorsum of the wrist afforded only temporary relief from pain. A division of the right sympathetic chain was carried out below the third thoracic ganglion and the upper segment was mobilized and buried in the anterior scalenus muscle according to Telford's technic. There was an immediate warming of the hand and an alleviation of all of his complaints. He used the hand quite freely but experienced a sharp twinge of pain whenever the wrist was strongly dorsiflexed. Within a few weeks of his operation he returned to work, but a short time later he bumped the back of his wrist against the steering wheel and his pain returned. Again it was necessary to immobilize the wrist on a splint. In spite of the fact that the hand was still warm and dry, the constant ache and burning seemed to be as bad as it was originally. Exploration of the wrist disclosed the presence of a small neuroma, little bigger than a match head, directly beneath the point of greatest tenderness. The removal of this neuroma resulted in a cure that was still complete at the end of a year of observation.

In view of these several considerations I believe it should be clear that neither of the alternative explanations offered to account for the cure of the causalgic states by a sympathetic ganglionectomy, can be considered to be entirely satisfactory. There must be a third alternative, some unknown factor that does not represent a simple release of vasomotor tonus or the cutting of a pain pathway. In seeking for a clue as to what this unknown alternative may be, one might start by abandoning, for the time being, the assumption that the activities of the sympathetic nerves represent the essential factor in either the cause or the cure of the causalgic syndrome. This assumption, so commonly made because the cure follows a procedure directed at the sympathetic pathways, may have obscured the evidence of a more fundamental disturbance involving the central nervous system.

There is plenty of evidence to suggest that the dysfunction of the sympathetic nerves is but one part of a more profound alteration of the physiologic status of the spinal cord centers. An outstanding example of this is the change that occurs in the skeletal muscles. Muscle weakness, incoordination, involuntary movements, contractures, etc., are recorded over and over again in the clinical records of these cases. The changes in function of skeletal muscle cannot be ascribed to the sympathetic nerves. Instead, they suggest that the anterior horn cells are being activated by the same central process that affects the cells of the lateral horn. There is evidence, too, in the distortion of sensory experience that characterizes the causalgic states, that the posterior horn cells may be involved in the same fundamental process. In fact, when one thinks back to the early stages of the causalgic state, and realizes that pain was the first and most outstanding of the symptoms, appearing before there is evidence of an involvement of the sympathetics or the skeletal muscles, it seems probable that the cells of the posterior horn of gray matter of the spinal cord were the first to be implicated in the central disturbance.

With these considerations in mind, it might be possible to reconstruct the chain of events that occurs in a case of causalgia, somewhat as follows: A partial lesion of a sensory nerve exposes bare fibers to scar compression or some other form of stimulation so that it becomes a focus of irritation; the sustained barrage of impulses from this focus acting on the internuncial pool of neurons in the cord, serves to disturb its normal functioning; the shunting of incoming impulses is altered so that the pattern of excitation, eventually registering in consciousness, is changed; the continued activity within the pool plays on the motor cells of both the anterior and lateral horns of gray matter; the muscle spasm and vasomotor abnormalities which result, lead to peripheral changes that furnish new sources for pain impulses; and, finally, as the intensity of this self-sustaining process increases, other systems of integrated neurons within the central nervous system are drawn into the process. I shall develop this concept in the next chapter, but I wish to convey, here, my impression of the sympathetic nerves as a part of a more fundamental central disturbance.

Evidently the part played by the sympathetic nerves is an important one, otherwise an interruption of their activities would not succeed in curing the causalgic state as often as it does. I do not know how the sympathetics contribute to causalgic states, nor how it happens that a periarterial sympathectomy, a ganglionectomy or even a temporary interruption of their functions by novocaine injection, may act to terminate the syndrome. It is possible, even probable, that the vasomotor activities of the sympathetic nerves play an important role in the maintenance and the cure of the causalgic state. That is to say, the sympathetic nerves may contribute to the development of peripheral tissue changes, which may lead to additional afferent impulses adding themselves to those from the trigger point to assail the spinal cord centers. This is not equivalent to saying that the sympathetic dysfunction *causes* the causalgic syndrome. It would be more correct to say that the trigger point *caused* it, but I believe that neither statement is wholly true. Instead, the trigger point starts the central disturbance, the central process in its turn involves the sympathetic nerves and the somatic motor nerves, and the peripheral effects brought about by the motor activity of each, initiate afferent impulses which add themselves to those from the trigger point to sustain and augment the central activity. The sympathetic nerve activity is but one part of this vicious circle.

The principal reason why I hesitate to accept either the trigger point or the sympathetic nerves as the sole *cause* of the causalgic state, is that either one of them may be eliminated without establishing a cure. I believe that the syndrome is cured only when the underlying pathologic activity *as a whole,* loses its momentum. Sometimes the syndrome may be cured by the removal of the trigger point without doing anything to the sympathetic nerves; sometimes the elimination of the sympathetic influence results in a cure even though the trigger point is left untreated; but in both of these events the *cure,* that is, the complete disappearance of the signs and symptoms, does not occur until the central process has subsided.

This interpretation of the relationship of the sympathetic nerves to the causalgic states is not an explanation. It answers none of the fundamental questions as to what these nerves do to the peripheral tissues to help maintain the syndrome. Yet it seems to me to be necessitated by the clinical observations. Without some such interpretation as this I find it impossible to adequately account for the cures that may follow the resection of an obliterated segment of artery, a periarterial sympathectomy or a novocaine injection of the ganglia. I know that the operations on the artery cannot sever any large number of either afferent or efferent nerve fibers, yet I am convinced that cures may sometimes follow these procedures. I have no reason to think that the local anesthetic effect of novocaine on the sympathetic ganglion cells lasts more than a few hours, yet I am convinced that cures are established by this temporary interruption of sympathetic influences.

The interpretation has afforded me a new approach to other

clinical problems than the ones under discussion, and a new attitude toward treatment. I am beginning to feel that the central disturbance is the essential factor in many diseases, and that there should be better means for eliminating pain than by a chordotomy or posterior root section or other *anatomic* interruptions of nerve continuity. I do not wish to venture too far into speculations regarding other clinical entities than those with which the monograph is chiefly concerned, but to make this point, I will make brief mention of two observations, one relating to deep venous thrombosis, the other to Hirschsprung's disease, both of which seem to lend themselves particularly well to the interpretation I am developing.

Leriche [66] suggested that the signs and symptoms due to a deep venous thrombosis respond well to repeated injections of novocaine in the sympathetic ganglia related to the involved limb. Ochsner and DeBakey [93] have more recently popularized the method in this country. Sometimes, after a single injection there occurs a startling change in the clinical course of the case. The edema diminishes, pain disappears, sweating moderates, the limb loses its discoloration and coldness, and the fever drops. Many of these changes are apparent within the first twenty-four hours after the injection, and in some instances a single treatment will modify the whole course of the syndrome. More often than not, the signs and symptoms do not disappear entirely, or they recur, so that more than one injection is required. Ochsner believes that the edema and its concomitant phenomena are ascribable to a spasm of the arteries which is brought about by reflexes from the thrombosed vein. He attributes the benefit conferred by the novocaine infiltration to a release of the arteries from vasospasm.

I have no doubt that Ochsner is correct in assuming that arterial spasm plays an important role in this syndrome. I am aware of the susceptibility of arteries to reflex spasm. I have examined the autopsy findings in two cases, each of whom died as a result of gangrenous changes in an extremity. In both cases, before the gangrenous changes became apparent, there had occurred a sudden cessation of all arterial pulsations in the extremity, as if the major arteries had been completely occluded. At autopsy no organic change was found in the arteries. The only demonstrable lesion was a thrombus in the femoral vein. Presumably the arterial spasm in these cases was initiated by impulses from the vein. I have seen extensive arterial spasm following injuries that did not directly involve the artery, and I know of one patient who has a tender place on his heel, which when pressed upon, will cause an immediate cessation of the arterial pulsations of the entire extremity. And I am sure that arterial spasm plays an important part in the syndrome of deep venous thrombosis. I do not know that arterial spasm causes the edema, but I am not making an issue of this question now. I am concerned only with the remarkable fact that a temporary block of the sympathetic impulses can bring about such striking changes in the physiologic status of the affected extremity. Nothing has been done to remove the pathologic impulses from the thrombosed vein, yet a single injection of novocaine produces a prompt restoration of a normal physiology that may remain permanent. And if the abnormal status recurs, repeated injections may establish a cure.

I have used this method of treatment for deep venous thrombosis. It is difficult to evaluate my results because I do not know what course these treated cases might have followed if the novocaine injections had not been carried out. Yet I am convinced that the method is capable of hastening recovery in many instances and lessening the chances of a persistent edema. I have been asked by other surgeons why I did not inject the sympathetic ganglia with alcohol, as I do in many cases of peripheral vascular occlusion. They point out that a longer lasting interruption of sympathetic influences might obviate the necessity for repeated novocaine injections. I find it difficult to answer their question. I have used alcohol a few times, and have felt that perhaps it saved the patient the discomfort of an additional injection or two. I do not feel that alcohol injection in the lumbar region is particularly hazardous, but the undesirable sequelae are greater than after simple novocaine injection. Certainly, I feel that if a "physiologic" interruption of the sympathetic influences can accomplish results that compare at all favorably with those obtained by alcohol injection, or a surgical excision of the lumbar ganglia, I would much prefer the former method.

The method of treatment and its end-results are of less importance, in my mind, than the implications to be drawn from these clinical observations. Presumably the syndrome is initiated by impulses from the thrombosed vein, which, in this instance, can be looked upon as the trigger point. The outward manifestations of the syndrome apparently are attributable to impulses conducted by the lumbar sympathetic pathways. The vasospasm, swelling and the nutritive changes which follow, furnish new sources for pain and new reflexes, so that a vicious circle is established. In some instances, left untreated, the process continues until permanent changes occur in the tissues and the patient is left with an edematous leg for the rest of his life.

If we are dealing here with a simple reflex from the irritant focus in the vein, to the artery, it might be anticipated that while the novocaine effect lasted, there would be a release from vasospasm and a temporary alleviation of the signs and symptoms. But it does not seem reasonable that the change should persist. The irritant focus has not been removed, and one

would expect that as soon as the blockade of sympathetic influences wore off, the clinical manifestations of the syndrome
would recur. Yet in many cases, they do not recur. And for
those in which they do return, subsequent novocaine injections
may establish a normal physiologic status which is persistent.

In my mind, the interpretation of these observations is essentially similar to that suggested for the causalgic states. And in
both interpretations the underlying factor of prime importance
is the central disturbance. The sympathetic outflow is important in that it maintains the disturbed function of the peripheral tissues. The irritant focus is important in the sense that it
initiates the process and tends to sustain or reactivate the whole
mechanism. But once the central process is started it assumes
the major role. It is the internuncial activity that must be restored to a normal equilibrium before a permanent cure is
established.

The second clinical observation that seems to me difficult to
explain, unless some central process is affected by the treatment, relates to Hirschsprung's disease. Scott [104] and Telford [115]
have each recommended the repeated induction of a spinal
anesthesia in the treatment of the moderately advanced case
of congenital megacolon. They have found in repeated instances, that a patient who had never had a normal ability to
evacuate the large bowel, may acquire this ability after the
administration of a spinal anesthetic. Spontaneous bowel movements may continue for a number of days or weeks after a
single injection. In the course of time the spontaneous function may fade, and again a spinal anesthetic restores it. A year
ago I gave a spinal anesthetic to a 48-year-old woman who had
a megacolon and a most distressing story of obstinate consti-
pation all her life. She was not cured by it, but at the end of
five months, she reported that in this interval she had had

more spontaneous bowel movements than in the previous forty-eight years. This may have been exaggerated, but a definite change in bowel function followed this single spinal anesthetic.

What possible effect can such an injection have on an atonic megacolon to permit it to function in a reasonably normal fashion for the first time in her life? One might say that the anesthetic temporarily suppressed an abnormally strong sympathetic influence exerted on the large bowel, which had prevented the parasympathetic "emptying mechanism" from acting. I should accept this explanation as adequate to cover the facts, if the patient had had a single involuntary evacuation of the bowel while still under the influence of the spinal anesthetic. But this is not what happened. She was considerably upset by the procedure and for three days nothing happened. Then she began having spontaneous evacuations. For several months these continued in quite a normal fashion. At the present time much of her improvement has been lost, but she still retains a better function than before the spinal anesthetic.

It is known that novocaine solutions within the dura may cause damage to the spinal cord and its nerves, so that one must be reserved in expressing the opinion that the result is not due to organic changes involving the sympathetic preganglionic fibers. On the other hand, there is no evidence to indicate that sympathetic function has been abolished. The observations suggest that a normal emptying mechanism may be present in Hirschsprung's disease; that it is held in check by some overactivity of the sympathetic influences, or prevented from expressing itself normally by some dysfuncton of the regulatory centers. One might say that the temporary effect of the spinal anesthetic "broke the vicious circle," or, better, that it produced some effect on the regulatory neuron systems, that restored normal function.

## CHAPTER XV

## The Vicious Circle

Webster defines a "vicious circle" as "A chain of morbid processes in which a primary disorder leads to a second, which in turn aggravates the first one." The origin of the term as it is used in medical terminology is obscure, but it has been in use a long time, and the concept which it embodies appears in early writings relating to the causalgic states. Mitchell[85] (p. 193) said: "Nerve injuries may also cause pain which, owing to inexplicable reflex transfers in the centres, may be felt in remote tissues outside of the region which is tributary to the wounded nerve. When the later pathological changes of an irritative nature which follow nerve injuries begin to occur, new causes of pain arise, the reflex references become wider, and when in certain cases the nutrition of the skin suffers, novel forms of suffering spring up, which are due to alterations of the peripheral nerve ends or their protective tissues." Bowlby[9] (p. 350) in commenting on nerve-stretching in the treatment of phantom limb pain, wrote in 1889: "Moreover, I can well conceive that if any nerve center be, so to say, broken of a vicious habit for a time, permanent cure may result even after reunion of the nerve fibers."

The concept has been utilized to account for the factors that sustain hypertension, certain skin diseases, "circus movements" in heart muscle, the progress of surgical shock, and many other clinical conditions. Exactly what the concept is meant to convey to the reader is not always made clear, but in general it conveys the impression of a series of interrelated events leading to a state of pathologic physiology which tends to become self-sustaining. The usefulness of the concept lies in the fact that if the sustaining factors are actually interdependent, the whole syndrome may be terminated by an attack on the point of least resistance. Hurry [56] wrote extensively on this subject in order to show how different disease processes might be cured by "breaking the vicious circle." Clifford Allbutt [4] wrote a review of Hurry's book, "Vicious Circles in Disease," and his comments contain so many ideas that are directly applicable to the concept I wish to develop, that I am quoting rather extensively from the review.

"A few days before this volume was placed in the hands of the reviewer he had been watching for a few minutes the race of a small brook into a larger but more sluggish stream. Curiously, near the inrush, a wisp of straws lay almost at rest, circling slowly round and round, but not swept with other wisps and leaves into the main current. This arrest was due to a still, but deep whirlpool, formed by the different velocities of the waters at the angle of meeting. Light objects which skirted this eddy swiftly vanished on their way to the sea; those caught in it were imprisoned. However, by placing a walking stick tangentially to the eddy, now one straw, now another, would dart aside, and, catching a streak of the main current, would speed off into liberty.

"This humble little parable may serve to illustrate Dr. Hurry's interesting volume on vicious circles of disease. The author's message may be summed up thus: In health the confluent or congruent streams of energy should work in a reciprocal harmony for the several ends of the organism as a whole; but in disorder, this agent or that, alien or home-grown, may strike tangentially upon one or more of such streams and form a vortex, twisting the lines of function and setting up, in one or more situations, a focus of wasting energy. . . . To disperse a vortex, expending energy in mere friction, may serve even to disperse the malady; at least it may moderate its intensity, or dispel vexatious symptoms. . . . There is one more demur. Dr. Hurry seems scarcely to realize, or fully to impress on us, the factor of 'organic memory' in these phases of function, the bent of biological matter to repeat what it has done before; a faculty on which development and purpose depend. In vicious circles every gyration deepens the groove, an abnormal habit is formed, so that arrest of such a local waste of energy and such a distress becomes more and more difficult; herein enters the problem of 'faith healing,' of the stronger tangential force which is to dissipate the vortex and redistribute the currents of energy. The longer the 'habit'—the fixture of organic memory—the harder the impulse needed to 'break the circle,' for the habit has become independent of the original cause, which indeed had often vanished."

The vicious circle concept, and many of the illuminating figures of speech employed by Allbutt in his review, seem to me to be applicable to the causalgic states. The sequence of events, as I interpret them, may be something like the following:

An organic lesion at the periphery, involving sensory nerve filaments, may become a source of chronic irritation. Afferent impulses from this "trigger point" eventually create an abnormal state of activity in the internuncial neuron centers of the spinal cord gray matter. The internuncial disturbance in turn is reflected in an abnormal motor response from both the lateral and anterior horn neurons of one or more segments of the cord. The muscle spasm, vasomotor changes, and other effects which this central perturbation of function brings about in the peripheral tissues, may furnish new sources for pain and new reflexes. A vicious circle of activity is created. If the trigger point is removed early, the process may subside spontaneously. If the process is permitted to continue, it spreads to involve new areas, and tends to acquire a momentum that is increasingly difficult to displace. Perhaps in this stage, even a removal of the original irritant may not be sufficient to establish a cure. But if an important part of the circle of reflexes can be interrupted, the process may subside, and a normal physiologic status is again established. If again the pathologic patterns gain the ascendancy, the repeated breaking of the circle may result in a permanent cure.

When I speak of "breaking the vicious circle" I do not have in mind a simple chain which becomes functionless when one link is broken. The process that underlies the cases I have studied has a more dynamic character than this. The cases are rarely "cured" by the first treatment, although such instances do occur. More often the immediate period of relief lasts but a few hours and is followed by a definite exacerbation of the signs and symptoms. In the favorable case, the exacerbation is followed by a secondary period of distinct relief, and as treatment progresses, the periods of relief become longer and longer, until the signs and symptoms are completely dissipated. In terms of the illustration of the vortex and the walking stick, one might say that the stick thrust into a strong vortex seemed to merely cause the whirlpool to churn more wildly, but each thrust, after its immediate turbulent effects had vanished, acted to gradually dispel the vortex.

If I were to undertake to translate this clinical interpretation into physiologic terms I would say that there were three reciprocating factors in the vicious circle of the causalgic state: incoming impulses from the periphery; the internuncial pool activity; and the motor impulses from the lateral and anterior horn cells that are brought within the influence of the pool. If one of the three interdependent factors could be said to be more important than the other two, I would select the internuncial pool as that one. It is the receiving station within the central nervous system which determines the routing of sensory impulses, and the dispersal of motor impulses to the periphery. Usually the status of the pool activity is such as to insure that the sensations which register in consciousness, and the patterns of motor response to stimuli, will be "normal." But when the pool is continuously bombarded by powerful impulses from a focus of irritation, its activities are disturbed so that there occurs a change in the routing of sensory impulses and in the patterns of motor response. One might say that the internuncial pool had become a whirlpool. At least, this term expresses something of my impression of a dynamic force within the central nervous system that gathers momentum and leads to destructive side-effects. It serves also, to illustrate a number of other clinical observations; how the disturbance at a given level may draw into its powerful vortex, other neighboring or even distant neuron systems; why the abnormal patterns of response may continue after the causative lesion has been eliminated; and the importance of an early attack before the destructive agency has acquired too great a momentum.

Such an interpretation constitutes an unwarranted extension of the physiologist's use of the internuncial pool concept. There is no experimental evidence to indicate that the activities of this neuron system can be changed into a "whirlpool." Furthermore, even though the activity in the internuncial pool may be self-sustaining and self-reëxciting in a closed-chain type of neuron relationship, the time factor measuring the interval of sustained activity is extremely short. It is expressed in millisecond units, instead of the minutes, hours and months that measure the persistence of clinical states. But if a single "conditioning" volley is capable of changing the fate of the "testing" volley in the laboratory, there should be no insurmountable obstacle to believing that reiterated impulses of pathologic intensity, maintained over a long period of time, might seriously disrupt the activities of the internuncial pool for a correspondingly long time.

Incidentally, certain recent experimental evidence suggests that internuncial activity set up by a single stimulus may continue for remarkably long periods of time, that is, remarkably long in comparison to the milliseconds and fractions of milliseconds that measure the activity of single neurons. Hoefer and Putnam [55] have made some interesting observations which illustrate this point. Recording electromyograms in cases of spastic paralysis, they noted that a single stretch stimulus might elicit a rhythmic sequence of discharges in the muscle that might last well over two-thirds of a second. Thus a record from the calf muscle would show the irregular spike discharge

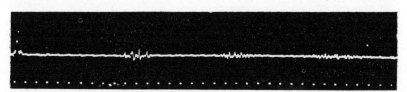

Fig. 26.—Electromyograms of Ankle Jerk Taken from the Calf Muscle in a Case of "Spastic" Paralysis

The irregular spike pattern of the primary response, at the left of the record, does not show clearly, but the rhythmic "clonic" discharges are shown well as three separate oscillations of diminishing amplitude. (Courtesy, Paul Hoefer.)

that characterizes the spastic case; then after a considerable delay, there would be recorded a second group of spikes of low amplitude (this time with no actual movement of the muscle); then another period during which no electrical changes would record; and then a third group of spikes of still lower amplitude. Their records indicated that the impulses set up within the internuncial pool by a single stimulus, had reached the motor horn cells in the expected manner, and then had disappeared into some "delaying path," only to reappear at the motor horn again, and yet again, as their mysterious circling activity was repeated. The observations of Hoefer and Putnam were interpreted as showing that in spastic paralysis, there was not only a change in the character of the motor response from the anterior horn cells, but also a loss of some inhibiting force normally exerted by the corticospinal neurons, which resulted in an abnormal spread of impulses within the spinal cord, and a repetitive circling of impulses within its neuron systems.

An even more mysterious observation of delayed response to a single stimulus, has been observed in relation to the "suppression bands" in the primate cortex, by Dusser de Barenne and McCulloch.[22] It has been shown that there exist several narrow strip zones bordering the principal functional areas of the cortex, which when stimulated, produce a suppression of activity in neighboring parts of the cortex. Thus the stimulation of the strip lying between the motor and premotor areas, will cause a rise in threshold of excitability of the motor cortex. Stimulation of a suppression band will also bring about a temporary disappearance of the spontaneous electrical activity of the cortex. A single stimulation will produce a suppression of electrical activity, not only of the adjacent cortex, but the wave of suppression sweeps over the entire cortex of both hemispheres simultaneously. The astonishing feature of these suppression effects is that they do not appear until many minutes after the single stimulation, and once established, they may persist for a half hour or longer.

These interesting experimental findings are not mentioned to justify my use of the internuncial pool concept, nor as having any bearing on the concept of a vicious circle of reflexes in clinical states. No one knows what the long-sustained suppression effects may mean in a physiologic sense, and it is most difficult to explain them in terms of neural transmission as it is understood today. They are mentioned only to illustrate the possibility that a single stimulus may set up activities within neuron systems that are sustained for much longer units of time than are ordinarily employed in measuring the activity of individual nerve units. As a matter of fact, there is no real necessity for demonstrating that a single stimulus can produce a sustained activity within the internuncial pool in such conditions as the causalgic states. In these states there is every reason to believe that impulses of abnormal intensity maintain a continuous barrage of influences that play upon the inter-related neuron systems within the central nervous system to sustain a functional disturbance.

Many everyday experiences suggest that activities set up within the central nervous system by long continued peripheral stimulation, tend to continue after the stimulus has been withdrawn. For instance, a man drives his car with the window open so that the wind blows strongly for hours across the hairs on the back of his hand. He reaches his destination and the stimulation of the hairs ceases, but he is aware of an uncomfortable feeling that there is something tickling the back of his hand. It feels like a cobweb and he tries to brush it off. The sensation persists, and after trying ineffectually to brush off the offending web, he examines the hand. There is nothing there. Yet for an hour or longer he continues to be annoyed by the illusive sensation. The sense of body vibration that continues after a long ride on the train, or the "sea-legs" of the man who comes ashore after a long trip at sea in a small boat, these and many other commonplace experiences illustrate the persistence of central activity after long-sustained stimulation.

It might be of value to compare the "concept of the vicious circle" as it is utilized by the psychiatrist to explain "tension states," with that which has been elaborated here in relation to the causalgic states. There is no need to detail the psychic irritants which may combine to suddenly precipitate the tension state. Nor is it necessary to point out that the development of visceral symptoms (palpitation, sweating, anorexia, etc.) and somatic symptoms (weakness, tremor, incoordination, etc.), combined with the emotional instability and other evidences of psychic perturbation, are all indications of a profound disturbance of the integrated neuron systems of the higher centers that regulate body function. The victim is transformed into a new individual, whose worry over his heart palpitation and other visceral dysfunctions, tends to add to his psychic state. There is thus set up a mutually augmenting and sustaining circle of activity that becomes increasingly difficult to displace. Even the removal of the original psychic irritants may not bring the individual back to normal. But if the removal of the psychic irritants is done early enough; if the patient is given a rational insight into the factors that precipitated the tension state; and if he can be assured that he has no organic disease, he may be restored to a normal equilibrium. And if, once again, the pathologic physiology of the nerve centers regains the ascendancy, the repeated breaking of the vicious circle may eventually establish a permanent cure.

There is a striking similarity between this central perturbation of function involving the higher centers, and that which I have assumed to involve the spinal cord centers in the causalgic states. In the one case, the irritants are psychic in origin;

in the other, they are organic lesions at the periphery. In fact, the two conditions are so much alike in their development, course, and response to treatment, as to suggest that the same kind of central disturbance of regulatory function may take place at any level of the central nervous system, and even to suggest that this is the characteristic response of functionally integrated neuron systems to chronic irritation.

Perhaps this is the most significant of the implications to be drawn from a study of the causalgic states. No one questions the fact that psychic irritants may set up an internuncial disturbance that acquires a momentum, which, unchecked, brings about, first a disturbance in function, and finally, organic changes in the body tissues. No one doubts that, by a psychiatric approach, it is possible to restore a normal equilibrium in the regulatory centers by removing the irritants or altering the patient's reaction to them. There can be no question that in some instances, this method of breaking the vicious circle restores normal function, and perhaps a reversal of actual pathologic changes in the tissues in the direction of normalcy.

Nor can it be doubted, that in some cases, the surgical removal, or medical cure, of internal disease, acts in a similar manner to break a vicious circle of reflexes that have been causing widespread dysfunctions, and perhaps organic changes in other organs of the body. But that similar, if not identical, dysfunction in the regulatory centers of the spinal cord and brain may be set up by peripheral irritants in the extremities, has not been so clearly recognized.

In making this distinction between the internuncial disturbances at different levels of the central nervous system, I do not intend to make an arbitrary separation of them, one from the other. I see no more reason for assuming that the causalgic states may not draw the higher centers into their circle of activity, than that psychic states cannot affect the spinal cord centers. In fact, I believe that no matter what the source of the irritation may be, the dysfunction may eventually spread to involve many of the functionally interrelated neuron groups of the entire central nervous system. The point which I would emphasize is that in the causalgic states, there is good evidence to indicate that the spinal centers are primarily involved, and the higher centers are drawn into the process secondarily, if at all.

It is difficult to find an apt comparison to illustrate the concept of the central nervous system that I would like to put into words. Suppose one were to think of the intricate interplay that normally takes place between the vast neuron systems of the central nervous system, as being called into activity in proper sequence in the same manner that a succession of harmonious sounds are produced from a phonograph record. The individual inflections of the instruments of a symphony orchestra that are woven together in the intricate pattern of sound, are no more complex than are the succession of muscular contractions and relaxations that enable the baseball pitcher to carry out a smooth wind-up and delivery of the ball. Let us imagine that the phonograph record is the agency by which this complex, but harmonious succession of muscle activities is called forth. Under normal conditions, with the needle in the groove, each neuron group is called into play in its proper sequence, and the result is a smooth and beautifully coordinated activity of the effector units. Suppose now, some disturbing factor is thrown into the mechanism which causes the needle to jump from its groove. The resultant activity is no longer integrated, nor can the needle, unassisted, get back into the groove again. The longer the needle stays out of the groove, the deeper will be the false path it cuts, and perhaps too, the greater will be the difficulty in getting it back into the normal groove and keeping it there. But if, before the false groove is cut too deeply, the needle can be lifted back into its normal groove, it may once more call forth the smooth and harmonious sequences which constitute normal physiologic activity.

# SUMMARY

There are no final conclusions to be drawn from this study of pain mechanisms in the causalgic states. The subject is too complex, and there are too many questions yet to be answered. This is a personal record of impressions derived from the work of many investigators and my own observation of pain syndromes over a period of years. They represent impressions rather than settled convictions.

On a few points only, I have what might be called convictions. I believe that the concept of "specificity" in the narrow sense in which it is sometimes used to identify sensory experiences with particular end-organs and nerve fibers, has led away from a true perspective. I am convinced that it is a mistake to assume that a certain pain syndrome must represent an "obsession," or be of purely "psychic" origin, simply because its manifestations do not conform to what we have been taught about the anatomy and physiology of peripheral nerve pathways. I believe that it is equally foolish to discredit the results of procedures, such as periarterial sympathectomy and novocaine injection, on the ground that their mode of action is obscure. I am convinced that the whole story of the causalgic states will not be learned from a study of the functions of the sympathetic nerves.

Beyond these few convictions, my impressions are still too plastic to be called conclusions. In formulating them for presentation, I have been burdened with the necessity of considering separately, subjects that are intimately interrelated, and

236

that sometimes represent different facets of the same problem. If this presentation leaves the impression that I am propounding a new theory, or advocating a particular method of treatment, then I have failed to say what I have wished to say. My intention has been to record my concept of pain in some of its psychologic and physiologic aspects; to interpret as well as I can the investigations of other men; and to present the only interpretations of the causalgic states that seem to me to fit the known facts.

Pain is a sensory experience that is subjective and individual; it frequently exceeds its protective function and becomes destructive. The impulses which subserve it are not pain, but merely a part of its underlying and alterable physical mechanisms. The neurons subserving pain probably represent more than one type. They are "specific" in the sense that they are "structures designed to lower the threshold of excitability for one type of stimulus and to heighten it for others." The neuron as a whole is to be considered the specific sensory unit, rather than its endings or its fiber. The specificity of function of neuron units cannot be safely transposed into terms of sensory experience.

Irritation of sensory nerves, particularly when sustained or excessive, is capable of initiating changes at the periphery and changes in the functional activity of neurons within the central nervous system, both of which act to modify the eventual pattern of excitation registering in consciousness. The phenomenon of hyperalgesia is probably dependent upon both peripheral and central changes that tend to modify the composite of impulses reaching the sensorium. Any distortion of the intraneural pattern of peripheral nerves may give rise to unpleasant or painful experiences during nerve regeneration. The phenomena of "protopathic" pain and hyperalgesia can be accounted for without the necessity for postulating the existence of special nerves.

A chronic irritation of sensory nerves may initiate clinical states that are characterized by pain and a spreading disturbance of function in both somatic and visceral structures. If such disturbances are permitted to continue, profound and perhaps unalterable organic changes may result in the affected part. In the causalgic states, the pain is but one expression of an abnormal internuncial activity. Both of the motor horns of the spinal cord are also involved, and in many instances the resultant muscle spasm and vasomotor changes can create new sources for pain, and additional sensory impulses of pathologic intensity which further contribute to the central dysfunction. A vicious circle is thus created.

There are different methods whereby the vicious circle may be broken. Posterior rhizotomy and anterolateral chordotomy may relieve pain, but these radical procedures should be used only as a last resort. The underlying process is a physiologic disturbance, and there should be better methods for correcting it than a permanent sacrifice of anatomical pathways. If done early enough, a simple removal of the trigger point may be sufficient to establish a cure. If this fails, a sympathetic ganglionectomy, or possibly some less drastic method of attack on the sympathetic pathways may be successful. Not infrequently, repeated novocaine injections of the trigger point, the sensory nerve pathways, or the sympathetic chain, may effect a cure. Any or all of these methods may fail, not because the choice of a point of attack is lacking in rationality, nor that the procedure fails to accomplish its projected end, but because the point of attack concerns only one part of the underlying mechanism that is sustaining the clinical state.

I have borrowed the concept of the "internuncial pool" from

the neurophysiologist in order to implement my interpretation of the nature of the central process which I believe is the essential factor in the vicious circle. Situated as this spinal receiving center is, disturbances of its function are reflected in a variety of peripheral changes, through the agency of the motor nerves, and perhaps of the sensory nerves as well. The perturbation of function starting in the internuncial pool, not only expresses itself peripherally, but may eventually involve other functionally related spinal and brain centers. Undoubtedly, in many of the causalgic states which have been long established, the higher centers become affected, and all manner of physiologic and even organic changes may take place in parts of the body far removed from the original focus of irritation.

Finally, it has seemed to me that the implications that can be drawn from a study of the causalgic states have a wider application than has been given them here. It may be that the process I have ascribed to the internuncial pool represents the characteristic response of all integrated neuron systems to sustained irritation. In causalgia the focus of irritation is represented by a somatic lesion, in the tension states it is represented by psychic irritants, while in angina pectoris it may be represented by an arteriosclerotic plaque in a coronary artery. Doubtless, in many clinical syndromes there may be a combination of somatic, visceral and psychic irritants, each contributing to the central process, whether they represent primary or secondary factors. Once a vicious circle is established, the process tends to become self-sustaining and it is increasingly difficult to stop. The activities of the regulatory centers within the spinal cord and brain, which normally are so beautifully synchronized, are thrown out of step with one another. If the irritant foci are removed early enough the central process subsides, the functional part of the syndrome is lost, and improvement becomes possible. If the process is permitted to continue for a long time, the habit pathways are cut deeper and it becomes more difficult to re-establish normal function, even after the original irritants are gone.

These concepts may be applicable to the treatment of poliomyelitis, peptic ulcer, neurovascular asthenia and many other clinical syndromes in which a functional element is recognizable in the symptom-complex. They may have a bearing on the interpretation of the variable results achieved by a surgical attack on hypertension and angina pectoris. They probably underlie the efforts that are being made to recognize and counteract the earliest signs of surgical shock or an increasing intracranial pressure, before the regulatory mechanisms are so seriously involved that a normal equilibrium is no longer attainable. The whole art of medicine tends to become increasingly scientific as its interpretations become physiologic, and in the search for the irritants that disturb the physiology of the regulatory centers of the central nervous system, the efforts of the surgeon, the internist, the psychiatrist, and the laboratory worker are drawn closer together in a common purpose.

# BIBLIOGRAPHY

1. ADRIAN, E. D.: *The Mechanism of Nervous Action*. Philadelphia, University of Pennsylvania Press, and London, Oxford University Press, 1932, 103 pp.
2. ———— Latest Contributions to Study of Sensory Mechanism of Nervous System, Fiziol. zhur., 19:405-410, 1935.
3. ANDERSON, R., LIVINGSTON, W. K. and Dow, R. S.: Effect of Chronic Painful Lesions on Dorsal Root Reflexes in the Dog, J. Neurophysiol., 4:427-429, 1941.
4. ALLBUTT, C.: Review of Vicious Circles in Disease by J. B. Hurry, Nature, 86:374, 1911.
5. BAILEY, A. A. and MOERSCH, F. P.: Phantom Limb Pain, Canadian M. A. J., 45:37-42, 1941.
6. BARD, P.: *MacLeod's Physiology in Modern Medicine* (pp. 1-200). St. Louis, C. V. Mosby Co., 1941, 1256 pp.
7. BLUEMEL, C. S.: *The Troubled Mind*. Baltimore, Williams and Wilkins, 1938, 520 pp.
8. BORING, E. G.: Cutaneous Sensation After Nerve Division, Quart. J. Exper. Physiol., 10:1-95, 1916.
9. BOWLBY, A. A.: *Injuries and Diseases of Nerves*. London, J. and A. Churchill, 1889, 510 pp.
10. BURGET, G. E. and LIVINGSTON, W. K.: The Pathway for Visceral Afferent Impulses from Forelimb of the Dog, Am. J. Physiol., 97:249-253, 1931.
11. CATTELL, McK. and HOAGLAND, H.: Response of Tactile Receptors to Intermittent Stimulation, J. Physiol., 72:392-404, 1931.
12. COGHILL, G. E.: The Structural Basis of the Integration of Behavior, Nat. Acad. Sci., 16:637-643, 1930. The Neuro-Embryonic Study of Behavior; Principles, Perspective and Aim. Science, 78:131-138, 1933. Growth of a Localized Functional Center in a Relatively Equipotential Nervous Organ, Arch. Neurol. and Psychiat., 30:1086-1091, 1933.
13. DALTON, P. P.: The Nature and Treatment of Certain Types of Referred Pain, Brit. J. Phys. Med., 2:155-158, 1939.
14. DANDY, W. E.: Concealed Ruptured Intervertebral Discs, J. A. M. A., 117:821-823, 1941.
15. ———— Trigeminal Neuralgia and Pains in the Face, J. Indiana M. A., 31:669-672, 1938.

16. Dandy, W. E.: Treatment of Trigeminal Neuralgia by Cerebellar Route, Ann. Surg., 96:787-795, 1932.

17. Davis, L. E.: The Pathway for Visceral Impulses within the Spinal Cord, Am. J. Physiol., 59:381-393, 1922.

18. DeTakats, G.: Reflex Dystrophy of the Extremities, Arch. Surg., 34:939-956, 1937.

19. Dogliotti, A. M.: Traitment des syndromes douloureux de la périphérie par l'alcoolisation sub-arachnoidienne des racines postérieures a leur emergence de la moelle speniere, Presse méd., 67:1249-1252, 1931.

20. Dunbar, H. F.: Emotion and Bodily Changes. New York, Columbia University Press, 1938, 601 pp.

21. Dusser de Barenne, J. G.: Die Strychninwirkung auf das Zentralnervensystem. IV. Mitteilung, Folia Neurobiol. 6:277-286, 1912.

22. Dusser de Barenne, J. G. and McCulloch, W. S.: Extinction; Local Stimulatory Activity in the Motor Cortex, Am. J. Physiol., 113:97-98, 1935. Factors for Facilitation and Extinction in the Central Nervous System, J. Neurophysiol. 2:319-355, 1939. Suppression of Motor Response upon Stimulation of Area 4-s of the Cerebral Cortex, Am. J. Physiol., 126:462, 1939.

23. Echlin, G. and Propper, N.: Sensitization by Injury of the Cutaneous Nerves in the Frog, J. Physiol., 88:388-400, 1937.

24. Editorial—"Pain and Disease", Brit. M. J., 1:340-341, 1938.

25. Fay, T.: Problems of Pain Reference to Extremities; Their Diagnosis and Treatment, Am. J. Surg., 44:52-63, 1939.

26. Flothow, P. G.: Therapeutic Considerations in Diseases and Conditions, Related to the Sympathetic Nerves, Encyclopedia of Med. Surg. & Spec., 14:651-667, 1940.

27. Foerster, O.: On the Indications and Results of the Excision of Posterior Spinal Roots in Man, Surg. Gynec. Obst., 16:463-474, 1913.

28. Foerster, O. and Gagel, O.: Die Vorderseitenstrangdurchschneidungbeim Menschen, Ztschr.f.d.ges. Neurol.u.Psychiat., 138:1-92, 1932.

29. ——— Uber afferents Nervenfasern in den vorderen Wurzeln, Ztschr.f.d.ges. Neurol.u.Psychiat., 144:313-324, 1933.

30. Foerster, O.: Du Leitungsbahen des Schmerzegefuhls und die Chirurgische Behandlung der Schmerzzustande. Berlin, Urban & Schwartzenberg, 1927, 360 pp.

31. Ford, F. R. and Wilkins, L.: Congenital Universal Insensitiveness to Pain, Bull. Johns Hopkins Hosp., 62:448-466, 1938.

32. FRAZIER, C. H., LEWY, F. H. and ROWE, S. N.: The Origin and Mechanism of Paroxysmal Neuralgic Pain and the Surgical Treatment of Central Pain, Brain, 60:44-51, 1937.

33. FREY, M. VON: Beiträge sur Sinnesphysiologie der Haut; 111 Ber.d.Konigl.sachs. Gesselsch.d. Wissl. Math-phys. Klin. Leipsig, 1895, Sitzung vom.4, Marz, 176-184.

34. ———— The Distribution of Afferent Nerves in the Skin, J.A.M.A., 47:645-648, 1906.

35. FULTON, J. F.: *Physiology of the Nervous System.* New York, Oxford Medical Publications, 1938, 675 pp.

36. ———— *Selected Readings in the History of Physiology,* Springfield, Charles Thomas, 1930, 317 pp.

37. GASSER, H. S.: Axons as Samples of Nervous Tissue, J. Neurophysiol., 2:361-369, 1939.

38. ———— Recruitment of Nerve Fibers, Am. J. Physiol., 121:193-202, 1938.

39. ———— Control of Excitation in the Nervous System, Bull. New York Acad. Med., 13:324-348, 1937, and *Harvey Lectures, 1937,* Lancaster, Pa., The Science Press, 1937.

40. ———— Conduction in Nerves in Relation to Fiber Types, A. Research Nerv. & Ment. Dis. Proc., 15:35-59, 1935.

41. GASSER, H. S. and GRUNDFEST, H.: Axon Diameters in Relation to Spike Dimensions and Conduction Velocity in Mammalian Fibers, Am. J. Physiol., 127:393-414, 1939.

42. GELLHORN, E., GELLHORN, H. and TRAINOR, J.: The Influence of Spinal Irradiations on Cutaneous Sensations. 1. The Localization of Pain and Touch Sensations Under Irradiation, Am. J. Physiol., 97:491-499, 1931.

43. GOLDSCHEIDER, A.: *Dielehre von den Specifischen Energieen der Sinnesorgane.* Berlin, L. Schumacher, 1881, 40 pp.

44. GOLDSCHEIDER, A. and BRUCKNER, A.: Zur physiologie des Schmertzes; Die sensibilitat der haut des Auges, Berlin Klin. Wchnschr., 16:1226, 1919.

45. HARRIS, W.: Recent Work on the Trigeminal Nerve, Lancet, 1:587-588, 1939.

46. HEAD, H.: *Studies in Neurology.* 2 vol. London, Oxford University Press, 1920, 862 pp.

47. HEAD, H., RIVERS, W. H. and SHERREN, J.: The Afferent Nervous System from a New Aspect, Brain, 28:99-115, 1905.

48. HEAD, H. and HOLMES, G.: Sensory Disturbances from Cerebral Lesions, Brain, 34:102-254, 1911–12.

49. HEAD, H. and THOMPSON, T.: The Grouping of Afferent Impulses within the Spinal Cord, Brain, 29:537-741, 1906.

50. HERINGA, G. C. and BOEKE, J.: Protopathic Sensibility of Skin, Nederl. Tijdschr.v. Geneesk., 1:4-12, 1925.

51. HERRICK, C. J.: An Introduction to Neurology. Philadelphia, W. B. Saunders Co., 2nd Ed., 1918, 394 pp.

52. HILTON, J.: Rest and Pain. London, Bell and Sons, 5th Ed., 1892, 514 pp.

53. HINSEY, J. C.: (personal communication).

54. HOMANS, J.: Minor Causalgia; A Hyperesthetic Neurovascular Syndrome, New England. J. Med., 222:870-874, 1940.

55. HOEFER, P. F. A. and PUTNAM, T. J.: Action Potentials of Muscles in "Spastic" Conditions, Arch. Neurol. Psychiat., 43:1-22, 1940.

56. HURRY, J. B.: Vicious Circles in Association with Diseases of the Skin, Brit. M. J., 2:1686-1690, 1911. The Breaking of the Vicious Circle, Brit. M. J., 1:274-276, 1913. Vicious Circles in Disease. London, J. and A. Churchill, 1911, 186 pp.

57. JUDOVITCH, B. D. and BATES, W.: Common Back Strain; Lumbo-Sacral Sprain with Secondary First Lumbar Neuralgia, Med. Rec., 143:96-98, 1936.

58. KARPLUS, J. P. and KREIDL, A. E.: Ein Beitrag zur Kenntnis der Schmerzleitung in Rückenmark, Pflueger's Arch.f.d.ges. Physiol., 158:275-287, 1914.

59. KELLGREN, J. H.: A Preliminary Account of Referred Pains Arising from Muscle, Brit. M. J., 1:325-327, 1938. Observations on Referred Pain Arising from Muscles, Clin. Sc., 3:175-190, 1938.

60. KILGORE, A.: Case Report; Discussion of Back Disabilities, West. J. Surg., 49:264, 1941.

61. LANGLEY, J. N.: The Autonomic Nervous System. Cambridge, Heffer, 1921, 80 pp.

62. LASHLEY, K. S.: The Thalamus and Emotion, Psychol. Rev., 45:42-61, 1938. Integrative Functions of the Cerebral Cortex, Physiol. Rev., 13:1-42, 1933.

63. —— Brain Mechanisms and Intelligence. University of Chicago Press, 1929, 186 pp. Factors Limiting Recovery After Central Nervous Lesions, J. Nerv. & Ment. Dis., 88:733-755, 1938. Functional Determinants of Cerebral Localization, Arch. Neurol. Psychiat., 38:371-387, 1937.

64. LERICHE, R.: The Surgery of Pain. Baltimore, Williams and Wilkins, 1939 (Translated by Archibald Young) 512 pp.

65. LERICHE, R., FONTAINE, R., and DUPERTUIS, S. M.: Arterectomy;

with Follow-up Studies on 78 Operations, Surg. Gynec. & Obst., **64**:149-156, 1937.

66. LERICHE, R. and KUNLIN, J.: Traitment immediat des phlébites post-opératoires par l'infiltration novocainique du sympathique lombaire, Presse Méd., **42**:1481-1482, 1934.

67. LEWIS, T.: Suggestions Relating to the Study of Somatic Pain, Brit. M. J., **1**:321-325, 1938.

68. —— *Pain.* New York, The Macmillan Company, 1942, 192 pp.

69. —— The Nocifensor System of Nerves and Its Reactions, Brit. M. J., **1**:431-435, 1937. Experiments Relating to Cutaneous Hyperalgesia and Its Spread Through Somatic Nerves, Clin. Sc., **2**:373-417, 1936. The Effect of Asphyxia and Cocaine on Nerves Belonging to the Nocifensor System, Clin. Sc., **3**:59-65, 1937.

70. LEWIS, T. and KELLGREN, J. H.: Observations Relating to Referred Pain, Visceromotor Reflexes and other Associated Phenomena, Clin. Sc., **4**:47-71, 1939.

71. LEWY, F. H. and GRANT, F. C.: Physiopathologic and Pathoanatomic Aspects of Major Trigeminal Neuralgia, Arch. Neurol. Psychiat., **40**:1126-1134, 1938.

72. LIVINGSTON, K. E.: (personal communication).

73. LIVINGSTON, W. K.: *The Clinical Aspects of Visceral Neurology.* Springfield, Charles Thomas, 1935, 254 pp.

74. —— Post-traumatic Pain Syndromes, West. J. Surg., **46**:341-347 and 426-434, 1938. Irritative Nerve Lesions, Confinia Neurologica, **3**:193-219, 1940.

75. —— Back Disabilities Due to Strain of the Multifidus Muscle, West. J. Surg., **49**:259-265, 1941.

76. —— Trigeminal Neuralgia, West. J. Surg., **48**:205-211, 1940.

77. —— Fantom Limb Pain, Arch. Surg., **37**:353-370, 1938.

78. McGREGOR, H. G.: *The Emotional Factor in Visceral Disease.* London, Oxford Press, 1938, 198 pp.

79. MAHONEY, C. S. DE GUTERRIEZ: Phantom Limb Pain Treated by Cortical Excision (paper read before Harvey Cushing Society, unpublished).

80. MAYERS, L. H. and LIVINGSTON, S. K.: The Treatment of Arthritis and Associated Conditions; A Preliminary Report, Indust. Med., **8**:3-23, 1939.

81. MEIGE, H. and BENISTY, A.: Lesions vasculaire associées aux blessures des nerfs périphériques, Rev. Neurol., Paris, **23**:631, 1916.

82. MITCHELL, J. K.: *Remote Consequences of Injuries of Nerves and Their Treatment.* Philadelphia, Lea Brothers and Co., 1895, 245 pp.

83. MITCHELL, S. W., MOREHOUSE, G. E. and KEEN, W. W.: *Gunshot Wounds and Other Injuries of Nerves.* Philadelphia, J. B. Lippincott, 1864, 164 pp.

84. —— Reflex Paralysis, Circular No. 6, Surgeon General's Office, Washington, D. C., March 10, 1864.

85. MITCHELL, S. W.: *Injuries of Nerves and Their Consequences.* Philadelphia, J. B. Lippincott Co., 1872, 377 pp.

86. MOLOTKOFF, A. G.: The Source of Pain in Amputation Stumps in Relation to the Rational Treatment, J. Bone & Joint Surg., 17:419-423, 1935.

87. MOORE, R. M.: Some Experimental Observations Relating to Visceral Pain, Surgery, 3:534-555, 1938.

88. MOORE, R. M. and SINGLETON, A. O., JR.: Studies on the Pain Sensibility of Arteries, Am. J. Physiol., 104:267-275, 1933.

89. MÜLLER, J.: *Ueber die Phantastischen Gesichterscheinungen.* Coblenz, Jacob Hölscher, 1862. *Zur Verleichenden Physiologie das Gesichtssinnes.* Leipsig, Cnobloch, 1826, 462 pp.

90. NAFE, J. P.: A Quantitate Theory of Feeling, J. Gen. Psychol., 2:199-211, 1929.

91. NAFE, J. P. and WAGONER, K. S.: The Sensitivity of the Cornea of the Eye, J. Psychol., 2:433-439, 1936. The Insensitivity of the Cornea to Heat and Pain Derived from High Temperatures, Am. J. Psychol., 49:631-649, 1938.

92. NIELSEN, J. M.: Disturbances of Body Scheme; Their Physiologic Mechanism, Bull. Los Angeles Neurol. Soc., 3:127-135, 1938.

93. OCHSNER, A. and DEBAKEY, M.: Thrombophlebitis, J. A. M. A., 114:117-123, 1940.

94. PARÉ, AMBROISE: *Les Ouvvres D'Ambroise Paré.* Paris, Gabriel Buon, 1598. (Histoire de defunct Roy Charles IX, 10th book, Chapter 41, p. 401.)

95. PARSON, J. H.: *An Introduction to the Theory of Perception,* London, Cambridge University Press, and New York, The Macmillan Company, 1927, 254 pp.

96. PENFIELD, W. and McNAUGHTON, F.: Dural Headache and Innervation of the Dura Mater, Arch. Psychiat., 44:43-75, 1940.

97. POCHIN, E. E.: Delay in Pain Perception in Tabes Dorsalis, Clin. Sc., 3:191-196, 1938.

98. POLLOCK, L. J. and DAVIS, L. E.: *Peripheral Nerve Injuries.* New York, Paul Hoeber, 1933, 673 pp.

99. RANSON, S. W.: *The Development of the Nervous System.* 3rd Ed., Philadelphia, W. B. Saunders Co., 425 pp.

100. REICHERT, F. L.: Buccal Neuralgia; Form of Atypical Facial Neuralgia of Sympathetic Origin, Arch. Surg., 41:473-486, 1940.

101. RIDDOCH, G.: Central Pain, Lancet, 1:1150-1156 and 1205-1209, 1938.

102. ———— Phantom Limbs and Body Shape, Brain, 64:197-222, 1941.

103. Ross, K.: Trigeminal Neuralgia and Disseminated Sclerosis, Australian M. J., 1:587-588, 1937.

104. SCOTT, W. J. M.: Present Status of the Sympathetic Nervous System, New York State J. Med., 36:1955-1960, 1936.

105. SHARPEY-SHÄFER, E. S.: Recovery After Severance of Cutaneous Nerves, Brain, 50:538-547, 1927.

106. SHEEHAN, D.: The Clinical Significance of the Nerve Endings in the Mesentery, Lancet, 1:409-410, 1938.

107. SHERRINGTON, C. S.: *The Integrative Action of the Nervous System*. New Haven, Yale University Press, 1920, 411 pp.

108. SCHUMAKER, H. B.: Unpublished paper dealing with Novocaine Blockade of the Lumbar Sympathetic Ganglia to Relieve Labor Pain. (To appear in Proc. Soc. Exper. Biol. & Med.)

109. SJÖQVIST, O.: Studies on Pain Conduction in the Trigeminal Nerve, Acta. Psychiat. et. Neurol. supp., 17:1-139, 1938.

110. SLAUGHTER, R. F.: Relief of Causalgia-like Pain in Isolated Extremity by Sympathectomy; Case Report, J. M. A. Georgia, 27:253-256, 1938.

111. STEINDLER, A.: The Interpretation of Sciatic Radiation and the Syndrome of Low-Back Pain, J. Bone & Joint Surg., 22:28-34, 1940.

112. STEINDLER, A. and LUCK, J. V.: Differential Diagnosis of Pain Low in the Back, J. A. M. A., 110:106-112, 1938.

113. STOOKEY, B.: Trigeminal Neuralgia, *Nelson's Loose-Leaf Surgery*. Vol. V., p. 550.

114. STOPFORD, J. S. B.: *Sensation and the Sensory Pathways*. London, Longmans, Green and Co., 1930, 148 pp.

115. TELFORD, E. D. and SIMMONS, H. T.: Treatment of Gastro-Intestinal Achalasia by Spinal Anesthesia, Brit. M. J., 2:1224-1226, 1939.

116. TINEL, J.: Causalgie du nerf median par blessure a la partie moyenne du bras; insuffisance de la sympathectomie periartérielle; guerison par la section du nerf au poignet, Rev. Neurol., Paris, 25:79-82, 1918.

117. TÖNNIES, J. F.: Reflex Discharge from the Spinal Cord over the Posterior Roots, J. Neurophysiol., 1:378-390, 1938.

118. TOWER, S. S.: Unit for Sensory Reception in Cornea, with Notes

on Nerve Impulses from Sclera, Iris and Lens, J. Neurophysiol., 3:486-500, 1940.

119. TROTTER, W. and DAVIES, H. M.: Experimental Studies in the Innervation of the Skin, J. Physiol., 38:134-246, 1909. The Peculiarities of Sensibility Found in Cutaneous Areas Supplied by Regenerative Nerves, J. f. Psychol.u. Neurol., 20:102-150, 1913.

120. WALSHE, F. M. R.: The Anatomy and Physiology of Cutaneous Sensibility: A Critical Review, Brain, 65:48-112, 1942.

121. WATERSTON, D.: Observations on Sensation. The Sensory Function of the Skin for Touch and Pain, J. Physiol., 77:251-257, 1933.

122. WEDDELL, G.: Multiple Innervation of Sensory Spots in Skin, J. Anat., 75:441-446, 1941.

123. ―――― Clinical Significance of Pattern of Cutaneous Innervation, Proc. Roy. Soc. Med., 34:776-778, 1941.

124. WEDDELL, G., GUTTMANN, L. and GUTTMANN, E.: Local Extension of Nerve Fibers into Denervated Areas of Skin, J. Neurol. Psychiat., 4:206-225, 1941.

125. WHITE, J. C. and SMITHWICK, R.: *The Autonomic Nervous System*. New York, The Macmillan Company, 1941, 469 pp.

126. WOLFF, H. G., HARDY, J. D. and GOODDELL, H.: Studies on Pain and Action of Analgesics, Tr. A. Am. Physicians, 54:325-328, 1939. Studies on Pain. A New Method for Measuring Pain Threshold; Observations on Spatial Summation of Pain, J. Clin. Investigation, 19:649-680, 1940. Measurement of the Effect on the Pain Threshold of Acetylsalicylic acid, Acetanilid, Acetphenetidin, Aminopyrine, Ethyl Alcohol, Trichlorethylene, A Barbiturate, Quinine, Ergotamine Tartrate and Caffeine: An Analysis of Their Relation to the Pain Experience, J. Clin. Investigation, 20:63-80, 1914. Studies in Pain: Analysis of Analgesic Action of Ethyl Alcohol, Tr. A. Am. Physicians, 56:317-320, 1941.

127. WOOLLARD, H. H.: Anatomy of Peripheral Sensation, Brit. M. J., 2:861-862, 1936.

128. ―――― Intradermal Nerve Endings, J. Anat., 71:54-60, 1936–37.

129. WOOLLARD, H. H., WEDDELL, G. and HARPMAN, J. A.: Observations on Neurohistological Basis of Cutaneous Pain, J. Anat., 74:413-440, 1940.

130. ZOTTERMAN, Y.: Pain, Touch and Tickling, J. Physiol., 95:1-28, 1939.

# INDEX